GW00771842

Neurosurgery
for
Basic Surgical Trainees
Second Edition

Neurosurgery
for
Basic Surgical Trainees
Second Edition

W. Adriaan Liebenberg
*MB ChB (Stellenbosch), MMed Neurochirurgie (Stellenbosch),
FC Neurosurg. (SA)*

and

Reuben D. Johnson
DPhil, FRCS (Neuro. Surg.)

Forewords by
Carl Hardwidge
BM, FRCS
and
Richard J. Stacey
MBBS, FRCS, FRCS (SN)

HIPPOCRATES BOOKS

2nd Edition
Copyright © Hippocrates Books, 2010
Box 15, Carnforth LA6 1HW, UK

All rights reserved. No part of this publication may be translated into other languages, reproduced, stored in a retrieval system, or transmitted, in any form or by any means, electronic, mechanical, photocopying, recording or otherwise, without the prior permission in writing of the publisher.

No responsibility or liability is assumed by either the authors or the publisher for any injury, loss, or damage to persons or property as a matter of products liability, negligence, or otherwise, or from the use or operation of any methods, products, instruments, instructions, or ideas contained in this book. Every effort has been made to ensure that the details given in this book regarding the choice, operation or use of any instrumentation, or the choice, dosage and administration practices relating to pharmaceutical agents, which are mentioned in the text, are in accordance with the recommendations and practices current at the time of publication. However, because new research constantly leads to such recommendations and practices being updated, the reader should obtain independent verification of diagnoses and check the makers' instructions carefully regarding the choice and use of instruments, and regarding the administration practices, doses, indications and contraindications associated with pharmaceutical agents, before using any of the instruments or pharmaceutical agents mentioned in this book.

The statements made, and the opinions expressed, in this book are those of the authors and do not necessarily reflect the views of the company or companies which manufacture and/or market any of the instruments or pharmaceutical products referred to, nor do any statements made amount to an endorsement of the quality or value of such instruments or products, or of any claims made by their manufacturers.

ISBN 978-0-9547314-1-0

1st Edition
Copyright © Hippocrates Books, 2004
ISBN-10 0-9547314-0-9
ISBN-13 978-0-9547314-0-3

Typeset by The Drawing Room Design Ltd., Over Kellet, Carnforth, Lancashire, UK
Printed in Great Britain by the MPG Books Group, Bodmin and King's Lynn

CONTENTS

FOREWORD TO THE FIRST EDITION

At the start, a Senior House Officer's job in neurosurgery is daunting; nevertheless I remember my first day with some degree of affection – after all, it started me on the first steps of my soon to be chosen career. I also remember the considerable anxiety I felt. It was lucky that I had an infinitely patient Senior Registrar who held my hand until I had gained sufficient knowledge and experience to become a useful member of the team. This book will not stop any sensible SHO or newly appointed Registrar from being anxious in his or her new job, but it will give them access to an infinitely patient Senior Registrar who has the advantage of being constantly accessible and fits into their white coat pocket. Liebenberg and Johnson have managed to produce a text that is a working man's guide to day-to-day practical neurosurgery. They have combined discursive passages with a quick guide, which allows instant access to the information needed to run a neurosurgical ward on a day-to-day basis. I congratulate them on their efforts. I believe this book will be standard equipment for the new SHO and Registrar in neurosurgery.

Carl Hardwidge BM, FRCS
Consultant Neurosurgeon
Hurstwood Park Neurological Centre
Haywards Heath, West Sussex, UK

FOREWORD TO THE SECOND EDITION

Although many changes have taken place in the way in which surgeons are trained, one thing at least has remained constant – the need of the trainee for a readily available source of authoritative, reliable and, above all, clear and unambiguous advice on the day-to-day practicalities of the job. *Neurosurgery for Basic Surgical Trainees* has served that purpose well for the past five years, during which time it has established itself as the essential companion for all neurosurgical trainees. This new edition is even better placed to undertake that role, the authors having drawn upon the extensive experience of many of their colleagues in revising, extending and updating the chapters, whilst at the same time retaining the solid foundation of common-sense advice that characterised the first edition and which was so reassuring to those entering this demanding surgical specialty.

The successful outcome of any operative procedure depends not only upon the skill of the neurosurgeon, but also upon the combined efforts of the nursing staff and other health care professionals who work in, or have dealings with, with the neurosurgical unit. Although this book is aimed primarily at neurosurgical trainees, the style of writing and the clear explanation of concepts and terminology make it eminently suitable for a much wider readership, and I have no doubt that it will prove invaluable to all who provide patient care and support before, during and after the surgical procedure.

The authors, and those others upon whose assistance the authors have called, are once again to be congratulated on having provided an invaluable (and admirably succinct!) guide to the essentials of managing neurosurgical patients.

Richard J. Stacey MBBS, FRCS, FRCS (SN)
Consultant Neurosurgeon
John Radcliffe Hospital,
Oxford, UK

PREFACE

The management of neurosurgical patients can appear complex and daunting to the junior surgical trainee. Unfortunately, due to reductions in junior doctors' hours resulting from training programme changes and as a result of the introduction of the European directive on working hours, there has been a dramatic reduction in training opportunities in the UK. The specific need that was already apparent when the first edition of this book was produced five years ago, for a pocket text that will guide the junior surgical trainee through the essentials of managing neurosurgical patients, has therefore become even more pressing.

This volume has been written specifically for the trainee starting their first neurosurgical post, and it is hoped that it will serve as a useful guide during the first few weeks of their job. The rudiments of a neurosurgical history and examination are covered, followed by an overview of the different types of neurosurgical patient and range of neuropathological conditions that the trainee will encounter. Advice and tips are given on the management of emergency admissions and elective neurosurgical patients. The basics of interpreting neurosurgical CT scans are described succinctly. The fundamentals of the more common and standard neurosurgical procedures are described – from burr-holes to trauma craniotomy, from external ventricular drains to ventriculoperitoneal shunts. An overview of the use of neuro-ICU is given and an approach to neuro-ICU patients outlined. To help trainees make the most of their time in neurosurgery, and to facilitate their discussions with senior colleagues, a chapter is included which overviews some of the controversies and evidence base in neurosurgery.

Our decision to undertake this second edition was prompted primarily by the overwhelmingly positive response to the first edition, a response which we have found truly humbling. In addition, we felt that certain changes and developments in the book were particularly needed. Although the first edition had been written with the British neurosurgical trainee specifically in mind, it was met with an astonishing degree of interest amongst their counterparts in many other countries, most notably the USA. Whilst in the new edition British terms such as Consultant and Registrar continue to be used, the chapters have in all other regards been constructed with all neurosurgical trainees in mind, and trainees elsewhere should find little difficulty in substituting the senior surgical grades as used in their own countries.

We have been exceptionally fortunate in enlisting the services of a number of colleagues to update and develop most of the chapters, and to add some new ones. There is, for example, an outstanding new chapter on neuro-intensive care by Adel Helmy from Cambridge, whilst Saurabh Sinha, who trained in Sheffield and Oxford, has contributed an excellent and comprehensive introduction to paediatric neurosurgery. Other new chapters include a survey of hydrocephalus and shunt systems, and we are particularly pleased to have been able to include an account of neuronavigation techniques which are redefining our surgical specialty. To all those who have contributed to the second edition we extend our warmest and heartfelt thanks.

We hope that this second edition will prove to be as useful and supportive to trainees as the first appears to have been. If experience so far is anything to go by, it may not be the last, and we shall, of course, be more than happy to receive comments for ways in which it might be developed and improved.

W. Adriaan Liebenberg and Reuben D. Johnson, 2010

ACKNOWLEDGEMENTS

We are indebted to Mr Jason Thompson from Spine, Navigation & Neuro Technologies at Medtronic for his constant support for this second edition. Without the support of Medtronic this edition would not have been possible. We are most grateful to all the new authors who have endeavoured to update the chapters to ensure that this volume may achieve the aim of being a useful guide to the new neurosurgical trainee.

W. Adriaan Liebenberg and Reuben D. Johnson, 2010

This second edition was supported by an educational grant from Medtronic

LIST OF CONTRIBUTORS

Jonathan G. Bull
*Department of Neurosurgery,
Great Ormond Street Hospital, 30 Guilford Street,
London WC1N 1EH, UK*

Adel Helmy
*Division of Neurosurgery, Clinical Neurosciences,
University of Cambridge, Addenbrookes Hospital, Hills Road,
Cambridge CB2 0QQ, UK*

Reuben D. Johnson
*Department of Neurosurgery, John Radcliffe Hospital,
Headley Way, Headington, Oxford, OX3 9DU, UK;
Exeter College, Oxford, UK*

Timothy Lawrence
*Department of Neurosurgery, John Radcliffe Hospital,
Headley Way, Headington, Oxford OX3 9DU, UK*

W. Adriaan Liebenberg
*Paarl Medi-Clinic, Berlyn Street, Noorder-Paarl 7646,
P.O. Box 7267, Noorder-Paarl 7623, South Africa*

Deb Roy
*Department of Neurosurgery, Birmingham Children's Hospital,
Steelhouse Lane, Birmingham B4 6NH, UK*

Saurabh Sinha
*Department of Neurosurgery, Sheffield Children's Hospital,
Western Bank, Sheffield S10 2TH, UK*

Jignesh Tailor
*Division of Neurosurgery, Clinical Neurosciences,
University of Cambridge, Addenbrookes Hospital, Hills Road,
Cambridge CB2 0QQ, UK*

Hammad Qureshi
*Department of Neurosurgery, Birmingham Children's Hospital,
Steelhouse Lane, Birmingham B4 6NH, UK*

Julian Woollard
*Department of Neurosurgery, The Royal London Hospital,
Whitechapel Road, Whitechapel, London E1 1BB, UK*

1

Duties and Responsibilities of the Junior Neurosurgical Trainee

Timothy Lawrence and Reuben D. Johnson

CONTENTS

Overview and general duties
Organization of the working day
Taking neurosurgical referrals
    Details of the referring team
    Patient details
    History
    Examination
    Management in the referring hospital
    Plan
    Write it down!

OVERVIEW AND GENERAL DUTIES

There have been changes in surgical training the world over; for the most part, junior posts in neurosurgery are filled by two groups of doctors. The first is the career neurosurgeon who will be a trainee who has successfully made it into a highly competitive neurosurgical training programme; the other is a trainee in another specialty who is rotating through neurosurgery as part of their training. Regardless of the trainee's career aspirations they will be exposed to an invaluable training environment. Trainees will leave the job having developed vital skills in caring, on the ward and in the neuro-intensive care unit (NICU), for complex patients with both surgical and medical problems. They will be exposed to some of the most exciting advances in medicine in a specialty that is rapidly developing with new technology and scientific discovery. Neurosurgical pathology is extremely diverse, and a good understanding of systemic disease in addition to that within the nervous system is vital. A well organized junior team will have plenty of opportunities to go to theatre and to outpatients, and it is in these two places that neurosurgery really comes to life. Theatre, the NICU and follow-up clinics will reveal what neurosurgery can really achieve.

The duties of the junior neurosurgical trainee consist primarily of taking care of the patients on the ward during the day and out of hours, as well as running the pre-op clinics. With neurosurgery Registrars spending a large amount of time operating on both elective and emergency cases, the safety and care of the patients on the ward is very much in the hands of the more junior trainee. Occasionally, when things are busy, it may be necessary to carry the Registrar's receiving bleep. This is an excellent opportunity to learn, and it allows insight into the heart of the emergency neurosurgical service. A small section on how to take neurosurgical referrals is included at the end of this chapter.

ORGANIZATION OF THE WORKING DAY

In most units, the day begins with a morning meeting similar to the trauma meeting in an orthopaedic unit. The format differs between units but usually will consist of the Specialist Trainee years 1–3 (ST1–3) and Registrar on-call overnight presenting new admissions and referrals. Both the ST1–3 and Registrar may be asked detailed questions by the Consultants on the history, examination and scans of the previous day's admissions and referrals. Questions usually follow on the management options. This is an excellent forum in which to learn about neurosurgery, and the opportunity should be taken to ask questions of the Consultants, especially on more controversial issues. It is worth presenting patients before presenting the scan, so as to allow others to diagnose and locate lesions on the basis of history and examination alone.

After the meeting, the morning round will probably begin on the NICU and this will be led by the neurosurgical Registrars and anaesthetic team. Often, the junior trainees will be expected to present formally the patients and their progress over the last 24 hours, allowing the Registrars to make decisions regarding further management. It is essential that the trainee understands what is happening and the management plans, as they will probably be bleeped during the day to deal with any problems. The juniors should write in the notes on the NICU round. Care should be taken to document the diagnosis, any surgery so far and number of days post-op, the neurological status (Glasgow Coma Scale [GCS] score, pupillary response, focal deficits), cardiorespiratory status (use of inotropes, type of respiratory support and percentage oxygen), evidence of any infection, and a management plan for the day. The management plan should be a clearly numbered list, e.g.: (1) computerized tomography (CT) scan tomorrow; (2) if no changes on CT, wean sedation and reassess neurology; (3) keep intracranial pressure (ICP) <20 mmHg until sedation weaned.

The round will progress to the ward and ideally the juniors should present each patient, i.e., name, age, diagnosis, procedure, and progress. Nursing staff should be given the opportunity to raise any issues. Checklists for each type of patient are given in the later chapter on the ward management of neurosurgical patients. However, it is worth bearing a few matters in mind at this point. It is essential to check wounds frequently for signs of infection or cerebrospinal fluid (CSF) leak. Obviously, blood results should be available for the round, and particular attention should be paid to reporting daily sodium levels for patients with subarachnoid haemorrhage (SAH) and for patients after pituitary surgery. For patients with tumours, steroids should be reviewed each day to ensure that there is a plan in place for their discontinuation. Patients are rarely discharged on steroids, though a small maintenance dose may be given to tumour patients until they are seen by the oncologist, or to pituitary patients until they are seen by the endocrinologist. We make no apologies for repeating the point: never allow a patient to leave the unit without a plan to stop their steroids, and for someone to check this at a suitable date. It is advisable to be up to date on histology results and know when they are due, and to ensure that there are dates for oncology or endocrinology review.

Following the round, the ward jobs tend to consist of ordering scans and referring patients back to their local hospitals. Some units allow letters to be dictated, whereas in others letters will have to be typed. It is best if the junior trainees can find an efficient way of organizing referrals back. Valuable information often goes missing, so, if possible, document the name of the Consultant who referred the patient to the neurosurgical unit early on. Letters to the local hospital should include a summary of the presentation, details of the procedure, progress so far, a brief note about expected prognosis, details of medication (including plans to stop steroids), and arrangements for follow-up. Remember that many tumour biopsies are taken in the neurosurgical unit to provide a diagnosis so that definitive treatment can be planned and administered elsewhere.

Once all the ward jobs have been completed (hopefully by mid-morning!) the rest of the day will consist of covering the ward and NICU, seeing any new admissions, theatre, or pre-op assessment. If there is no afternoon round by the Registrar on call, it might be useful to get together with your team before the end of office hours to check that all results are back and acted upon. Ensure that any scans ordered have been done and seen, and decisions made by the Registrar or Consultant. It is the responsibility of the person who signs the request form to make sure that the scans are reviewed – so if you sign it, make sure you see the scan and show it to someone who can make a decision.

Pre-op clinics are much the same as in other specialties. Assessments are made for fitness for surgery and relevant investigations organized. It is essential to ensure that anticoagulants and aspirin are discontinued in good time before most neurosurgical procedures. Most Consultants prefer patients to be off all forms of nonsteroidal anti-inflammatory drug (NSAID) at least a week prior to elective surgery, particularly for intradural procedures whether cranial or spinal. In neurosurgery, juniors generally do not carry their own receiving bleep, are not asked to go to the Accident and Emergency (A&E) department, and are usually only required to attend a few outpatient clinics. However, in some centres the job is extremely busy with hours stretching far beyond those quoted on the rota. The neurosurgical post demands a high level of responsibility and knowledge. The junior trainees form the basis on which a busy department can function safely and effectively. A good junior trainee will be aware of the complexity of disease in neurosurgical patients, how rapidly a patient's condition may deteriorate and how vital the junior doctors are to the successful care of their patients. It is essential that the junior trainees work as a team. This is the only way everyone will get a chance to carry the Registrar bleep or go to theatre. There is ample opportunity to get hands on drills!

TAKING NEUROSURGICAL REFERRALS

Taking neurosurgical referrals is unlike taking referrals in most other surgical specialties you will have worked in. You will not always be able to walk down to the A&E department to see what is going on, because frequently the patient will be miles away in another hospital. Despite this, you may find that, once you have been phoned, the person making the referral will assume you have taken over the care of the patient! There is also a widespread assumption among referring specialties that all you need is the scans.

Never accept a referral of the type: 'Have you seen Mr Thompson's scans? Are you going take him?' Assume that, in such cases, Mr Thompson has fixed dilated pupils, a massive diffuse head injury, a clam-shell thoracotomy (but no IV access), bilateral open femoral shaft fractures, and has not had any C–spine films. Whilst this may seem obvious, the importance of obtaining as much of the relevant information as possible at the time of the first call cannot be overemphasized. If the person referring can't answer all your questions, make sure they understand that advice can be given only when all the information is available Remember to be polite: neurosurgical cases can be quite frightening, especially to the uninitiated, and we can all forget things in a crisis. By all means look at the scans and present them to your Registrar, but make it clear that the referring team is gathering all the facts. The following is the minimum amount of information that should be obtained from the referring team. Don't accept anything less!

DETAILS OF THE REFERRING TEAM

Name of referring doctor
Contact number of referring doctor
Name of Consultant in charge in referring hospital
Name of referring hospital

It cannot be overemphasized how important these details are. It is all too easy to put the phone down after obtaining a great history only to find you don't know which hospital the patient is in! Beware the 5 p.m. referral. The referring doctor might be going off-duty. Make sure to ask and that you know the contact details of their replacement.

PATIENT DETAILS

Name	Age
Date of birth	Location (emergency department/ward)

Remember that A&E departments can be quite big. If a patient is comatose in A&E don't just assume they are in resuscitation!

HISTORY

Sequence of events	Past medical history
Drug history	Social history

Obtain a concise sequence of events and begin to formulate a picture in your mind as to what sort of pathology you might be dealing with (see Chapter 4, on history and examination). Tailor questions according to pathology; e.g., if the history sounds spinal make sure to enquire about sphincter control. When the history is equivocal always enquire regarding a history of trauma (e.g., subarachnoids can be traumatic as well as spontaneous). If there is trauma, are there any other injuries? In the case of the comatose patient ask about medically reversible causes (e.g., fits, blood sugar). Past medical history and drug history are very important. If someone has a tumour on their scan it is vital to know whether they have a known primary. Similarly, if someone has had an acute subdural haemorrhage (ASDH), it is useful to know that they have atrial fibrillation (AF) and are on warfarin. A brief social history should be obtained along the lines of an orthopaedic-type social history, including details about mobility, e.g., 'Mrs Jones lives in a warden-controlled residential home, uses two sticks to walk, but is otherwise independent and takes the bus to go shopping'.

EXAMINATION

Current GCS	Peripheral deficits
Any fluctuations in GCS	Reflexes
Pupils: size and reaction	Sphincters
Cranial nerve abnormalities	Observations (obs)

Certain parts of the GCS may be more relevant than others; e.g., best motor response (see Chapter 4, on history and examination). Always make sure, therefore, that the person referring can break down the GCS into all its components and ask them what they mean – do not accept 'E1V3M4'! You need to ask them to tell you in words what the eyes, speech, and motor response actually are. Ask about fluctuations in the GCS: it might be 13 but it also may keep dropping down to 5. Pupil size and reaction need to be documented even if the GCS is 15, as pupil dilatation due to tentorial herniation can occur in the awake patient. Deficits in cranial nerve territory and peripheral nervous system help localize pathology. Sphincter assessment again is necessary if a compressive spinal lesion is suspected. Always take a note of the obs to include pulse, blood pressure, haemoglobin oxygen saturation (sats) and temperature. Always be thinking about whether the examination is consistent with the history. For example, a history of fits and confusion does not necessarily fit with a GCS of 15.

MANAGEMENT IN THE REFERRING HOSPITAL

Location of patient
ABCs and advanced trauma life support (ATLS)
Investigations
Treatments
Most senior doctor/Consultant's opinion

Make sure you know or enquire about the location of the patient. Remember that at this stage you are only taking a referral and are not managing the patient. However, if it sounds as though the patient needs to be in a high-dependency area, then suggest that this is discussed in the referring hospital. Are you happy with the airway? If a patient has a GCS less than 8 suggest that the referring team needs to speak to the anaesthetist in their hospital as intubation might be appropriate. Don't insist dogmatically on intubation at this stage unless it is obvious that the patient will need transferring. Remember, the patient may have had a pre-terminal event and intubation may be entirely inappropriate. If there is a history of trauma, has the full ATLS protocol been carried out? Enquire about what investigations have been undertaken and what is being sent to you. For example, have the scans been sent? In trauma, have C-spine films been undertaken? If there is a suspected tumour, what investigations have been undertaken to hunt for a possible primary? Make sure you find out what treatments have been initiated in the referring hospital (e.g., steroids, mannitol).

PLAN

You should always discuss the plan before you put the phone down, and document it clearly on your referral card/book. This might be that you will discuss the case and scans with your Registrar or Consultant and get back to the referring team. However, it might be that the referring team initiates some further investigations or arranges for an anaesthetist to be involved.

WRITE IT DOWN!

You may have got it all down into the book first time, or you may have jotted notes on the first available piece of paper. Make sure you write it all down in the book before you hand it over to someone else. Your documentation may be the only evidence of the advice that you have given.

2
Overview of Neurosurgical Patients

Jonathan G. Bull

CONTENTS

INTRODUCTION

Neurosurgery, like other specialties, is divided into subgroups. It is helpful to have some understanding of these and hence to be aware of where the interests of the Consultants in your unit lie. Boundaries between subspecialities may appear arbitrary and there are often considerable degrees of overlap between them. In the past, an individual's practice would evolve during their Consultant career. Increasingly, as trainees undertake subspecialty fellowships, their practice is becoming more defined. In some units, for example, a surgeon's practice may be entirely spinal, not involving any intracranial work, and perhaps even demitting from general emergency on-call duties.

There have also been significant changes in the scope and nature of many surgical specialities. Neurosurgery is no exception, and surgeons now work very much within multidisciplinary teams. This aids decision making, typified by an epilepsy surgery service where a single surgeon requires a large team of neurologists, neurophysiologists, neuropsychologists and specialist nurses to ensure that the most appropriate patients are selected for surgical treatment.

This team approach has also developed in response to the evolution of new treatment modalities, particularly in vascular neurosurgery. The International Sub-Arachnoid Aneurysm Trial (ISAT) demonstrated significant benefits, in some cases, of endovascular coiling of an aneurysm over surgical clipping. Interventional neuroradiologists are fully involved in discussions over treatment of these patients, and in many units the majority of aneurysms will be treated by the neuroradiology team. Only the most challenging aneurysms remain for surgery and these are not appropriate for trainees; this has led to the need for trainees to undertake subspecialty fellowships.

VASCULAR NEUROSURGERY

Vascular neurosurgery, as discussed, remains one of the highest risk subspecialties. Typically, surgeons manage individuals with aneurysms presenting either with subarachnoid haemorrhage (SAH) or incidentally. This entails, most importantly, the nonoperative management of SAH, which is one of the commonest referrals. Treatment decisions are undertaken in conjunction with interventional neuroradiologists and investigation by computerized tomography (CT) angiogram and/or formal catheter angiogram (with or without coiling). Vascular abnormalities, such as arteriovenous malformations (AVMs) and dural arteriovenous fistulas may be managed by operative or interventional means. Increasingly, some cases are managed by stereotactic radiosurgeons. In addition, cases such as cavernomas may be managed through watchful waiting, the key role of the surgeon being to give reassurance and thought as to the correct time for treatment. Surgeons are also carrying out bypass surgery (external to internal carotid) and carotid procedures (endarterectomies).

PITUITARY NEUROSURGERY

This encompasses the surgical treatment of hormone-secreting pituitary adenomas in cases where medical therapy has failed, or of space-occupying non-hormone-producing adenomas with the aim of preventing blindness and of reducing compression of brain tissue. Surgery is typically undertaken trans-sphenoidally, through the nose and sphenoid sinus, although re-do operations may be through an intracranial approach. Pituitary work is undertaken through a multi-disciplinary team so that cases are reviewed with endocrinologists and specialist nurses. Typically, there will be pre- and post-operative reviews by the physicians to ensure appropriate hormonal supplementation

SKULL-BASE NEUROSURGERY

This is a specialty embracing the treatment of tumours of the clivus, dorsum sellae, cerebello-pontine angle, around the third ventricle, foramen magnum, and parasellar area. The skull-base subspecialty has evolved dramatically since the first successful resection of a vestibular schwannoma in Edinburgh in 1896. Procedures are frequently undertaken with the assistance of ENT surgeons (translabyrinthine approach). In addition, the subspecialty has seen some of its more straightforward workload treated by stereotactic radio-surgery. The cases that remain are more challenging, again necessitating subspecialty training. A large group of patients exists where the surgeons and patients elect for a watch-and-wait approach with often lengthy pre-op observation and post-op follow up.

SPINAL NEUROSURGERY

Spinal neurosurgery encompasses one of the largest groups of neurosurgical patients, and there is significant overlap with orthopaedic spinal neurosurgery. Spinal neurosurgeons deal with a large number and range of degenerative pathologies, decompressing the spinal cord and nerve roots by means of laminectomies, discectomies and foraminotomies posteriorly. Anterior approaches may be undertaken, commonly in the cervical spine and less so in the thoracic and lumbar spine, necessitating thoracotomy or laparotomy. Furthermore, in patients with spinal instability, fusion of the vertebral column with instrumentation is often necessary. This typically involves the insertion of metal plates and screws or wiring in the cervical spine. In the lumbar and thoracic spine, pedicle screw fixation or inter-body fusion techniques are employed. Complex spine procedures are often undertaken in rheumatoid patients and in patients with achondroplasia. In addition, spinal neurosurgeons may be involved in the treatment of developmental abnormalities and deformities of the spine, including scoliosis surgery.

PAEDIATRIC NEUROSURGERY

Paediatric neurosurgery is almost a completely separate specialty, and there are ongoing discussions as to whether there should be a separate exit examination in paediatric neurosurgery. Nonetheless, paediatric neurosurgeons treat pathologies similar to those in adult patients in addition to the developmental abnormalities seen in children (see Chapter 9, on paediatric neurosurgery). Specifically, cases associated with the spinal and cranial dysraphisms, CSF circulation problems, and oncology form the bulk of the work load. Some paediatric neurosurgeons undertake subspecialty work such as craniofacial work with plastic and maxillofacial surgeons. The number of purely paediatric surgeons is growing, but with few purely paediatric units. Typically, more surgeons may cover paediatric emergencies on call, which most commonly involve shunt problems, subsequently handing on specific cases for urgent, rather than emergency, treatment.

FUNCTIONAL NEUROSURGERY

Functional neurosurgery is a fascinating and rapidly evolving subspecialty. Surgeons working in this area undertake the surgical treatment of chronic pain, movement disorders, neuropsychiatric disorders and epilepsy. This is usually undertaken in association with neurophysiologists and neurologists. Preoperative planning for deep brain stimulaton procedures is complex, and the surgery may be undertaken with the patients awake during the stereotactic insertion of stimulators (depth electrodes). Follow-up and adjustment of the devices is often done by neurophysiologists and specialist nurses.

Intractable dysaesthetic pain following failed back surgery or trauma can be treated with spinal cord stimulators, posterior rhizotomies or stimulation/ablation of the periaquaductal grey area or areas of the thalamus. Functional neurosurgeons may also be involved in the placement of spinal cord stimulators to treat chronic pain, and of baclofen pumps to treat spasticity.

Neurosurgeons involved in the management of epilepsy patients will carry out procedures to place intracranial electrode grids to help establish an epileptic focus prior to any subsequent ablation or resection procedures. Epileptic patients may also be treated with vagal nerve stimulators and deep brain stimulation.

PAIN NEUROSURGERY

Some neurosurgeons treat neurovascular compression syndromes, such as trigeminal neuralgia and hypoglossal neuralgia. The key task is to determine which patients will benefit. Typically, surgery is considered once medical treatment has failed or when side-effects can no longer be tolerated. A variety of methods is used, ranging from short term local anaesthetic injections when patients are *in extremis*, to ablative procedures such as radiofrequency rhizotomies. Microvascular decompression surgery may be undertaken to treat trigeminal neuralgia, but this operation is often done by a general neurosurgeon.

TRAUMA NEUROSURGERY

Trauma neurosurgery, currently considered part of the role of the general neurosurgeon, is evolving, with large units having subspecialists who are interested in the nonoperative and postoperative management of patients. Patients with head injuries will be admitted and treated in the first few hours by a general neurosurgeon and, in such units, referred to the subspecialist. The use of intracranial pressure monitors and probes for cerebral oxygenation and temperature as well as microdialysis are aiding treatment development in this field. Trauma neurosurgery encompasses intracranial injuries, such as traumatic haemorrhage (subdural, extradural, intracerebral haematomas), and diffuse axonal injury, skull fractures and spinal trauma.

RADIOSURGERY

Oncologists and some neurosurgeons treat patients with external radiation. The Linac accelerator, which works with conventional radiation beams, and the Gamma knife (Cobalt 60 source), are two focused external radiation sources that can focus on a very small area of brain and have a minimal effect on surrounding structures. The scope of these treatments has extended to include treatment of vascular (arteriovenous) malformations (AVMs), small skull-base tumours, and also some cases of neuralgia such as trigeminal neuralgia where surgery is not appropriate or will not be tolerated. The time to determine successful effect is longer, with patients treated for AVMs having to wait up to 2 years for conclusions with regard to the treatment outcome.

ONCOLOGICAL NEUROSURGERY

Oncological neurosurgery is a large field and generally constitutes part of the general neurosurgical remit. However, there is an increasing demand for neurosurgeons who subspecialise in neuro-oncology. Neuro-oncological surgery involves biopsy and resection of tumours both of the spine and the brain. Neuro-onclogy is a multidisciplinary subspecialty and surgeons collaborate closely with oncologists in determining management of these patients. There are currently many avenues of research into the possibilities and methods of determining the nature of tumours from radiology alone, so as to diminish the need for biopsy and its attendant risks.

GENERAL NEUROSURGERY

The ambit of the general neurosurgeon is usually taken to include spinal, trauma, oncology, CSF diversion, posterior fossa and peripheral nerve surgery. Typically, most neurosurgeons will cover these cases on call but may hand on more complex cases subsequently. Most surgeons are now appointed with a subspecialty interest, providing general neurosurgery cover on call.

3
Neurosurgical Pathology
W. Adriaan Liebenberg

CONTENTS

Disorders of CSF flow
  Obstructive (noncommunicating) hydrocephalus
  Communicating hydrocephalus
  Normal pressure hydrocephalus
  Benign intracranial hypertension
  Causes of shunt failure
Congenital disorders presenting in adulthood
  Aqueduct stenosis
  Chiari malformations
    Chiari I
    Chiari II
  Intracranial infection
Spinal disorders
  Tumours
  Degenerative disease
  Infection
  Spinal cord syndromes
    Syndromes of the upper spinal cord
      Anterior spinal cord syndrome
      Central cord syndrome
      Bell's cruciate paralysis
    Syndromes of the lower spinal cord
      Conus medullaris syndrome
      Cauda equina syndrome
Peripheral nerve disorders

CRANIAL DISORDERS
MANIFESTATIONS OF CEREBRAL DISEASE

As neurosurgeons, we deal mostly with either compressive or destructive lesions. The history usually gives an accurate idea of the type of pathology involved, and this usually is indicated by the length of the history and the progression. Patients who have sudden acute episodes with associated headache and immediate deficit or loss of consciousness, have usually had a vascular type of incident, whereas people who present with progressive mental dysfunction, speech difficulties and progressive limb deficits, usually have a tumour of some description. Sometimes, patients present with seizures alone, and this is quite typical usually of low grade tumours, or arteriovenous malformation, although this is not exclusively true. When presented with a patient who has a history of dysfunction and has clinical signs on examination, it is important to localize the lesion to the part of the CNS from which it originates. Specific lobes of the brain have specific functions.

Frontal lobes

The frontal lobes are concerned with personality, the cortical control of micturition and conjugate eye movement. The main function of the frontal lobes, however, is motor function, and the whole motor strip is found in the posterior aspect of the frontal lobe, in front of the central sulcus. Penfield's homunculus demonstrates which part of the cortex is responsible for which part of the body. A lesion on the convexity on the lateral side will cause dysfunction of the facial muscles, whereas lesions parasagittally in midline will cause dysfunction of the legs. Speech is also controlled by the lower part of the motor strip, the so-called Broca's speech area, and lesions here result in an expressive dysphasia. Seizures are common with frontal lobe lesions.

Parietal lobes

The parietal lobes are quite small; located behind the central sulcus, they are mostly concerned with recording sensory information and spatial orientation. Speech is relayed *via* the supramarginal and angular gyri. The other important part of the parietal lobes is the visual association area, governing awareness of the images recorded in the occipital lobes. Lesions in the parietal lobes therefore lead to cortical sensory loss, dysphasia in a dominant hemisphere lesion (speech is usually located in a dominant hemisphere), and dyspraxia (inability to move limbs appropriately because of a loss of spatial orientation) in a nondominant hemisphere. A parietal lesion would also lead to a homonymous hemianopia or an attention hemianopia (see Chapter 4, on examination).

Occipital lobes

The occipital lobes are truly small and are mainly concerned with visual function. Lesions in the occipital lobe lead to blindness in the contralateral eye with sparing of the pupillary reflex, which, as we shall see, loops only as far back as the brainstem.

Temporal lobes

Once again, seizures are a large part of the manifestation of temporal lobe pathology, and, as we shall see, a contralateral upper quadrant hemianopia is seen when the fibres of Meyer's loop are affected. The centre for receptive speech discrimination – Wernicke's area – is located in the superior temporal gyrus, and lesions in this area lead to receptive dysphasia. Bilateral lesions in the temporal lobe can also cause memory deficit.

Summary

- *Frontal lobes*

Motor function	Speech
Micturition	Conjugate eye movements
Personality	Higher mental function

- *Parietal lobes*
  Sensory awareness
  Spatial awareness (nondominant hemisphere)
  Speech (dominant hemisphere)
  Visual tracts
- *Occiptal lobes*
  Vision
- *Temporal lobes*
  Vision
  Receptive speech

TYPES OF CENTRAL NERVOUS SYSTEM (CNS) PATHOLOGY

Having taken a full history and carried out a full examination, and having put the signs together and come to the conclusion that the patient has a cranial problem rather than a spinal problem, and then having localized the problem to a suspected lobe, we are now ready to do investigations on our patient. Once we have the results back from our investigation, we then have to put forward a differential diagnosis. This is impossible without understanding the pathology of the CNS. The main types of CNS pathology that concern neurosurgeons are: malignancy; infection; inflammation; vascular abnormalities; and abnormal CSF flow patterns.

Intracranial malignancy

There are many ways of classifying CNS tumours. Pathologically, these tumours can be classified according to cell type: e.g., glial tumours or tumours of neuroepithelial origin. However, it can be extremely useful to consider tumours according to their anatomical site of origin in the CNS. In the forebrain and cerebellum, there are tumours that are inside the parenchyma of the brain and tumours that are outside the parenchyma of the brain but still inside the cranium. The first group are known as intra-axial tumours and the second group of tumours are called extra-axial tumours. What follows here is a discussion of the types of tumour that most commonly occur in different parts of the intracranial compartment. This is not a dry and formal description of pathology *per se*. Rather, it is a more general discussion which aims to include some insights into the particular problems different tumours present to the patient and clinician. Spinal tumours are considered later.

Intra-axial tumours

The most common intra-axial tumours are metastatic tumours that have spread mostly from the lung in males and breast in females (but also from the skin, kidney, prostate). The second most common intra-axial tumours are glial cell tumours and are known as gliomas.

Metastatic tumours

Metastatic tumours are sometimes treated by surgical excision. However, they are frequently multiple, and treating the cerebral metastases does not remove the primary tumour. The exception is in patients with fully treated primary tumours and single superficial metastases; these patients are quite often offered surgery, plus adjuvant therapy. The main aim in patients with metastatic tumours is tissue diagnosis; chest X ray, breast examination in females, and computerized tomography (CT) scanning of the abdomen are indicated to try and find a more accessible lesion from which to obtain a tissue diagnosis. If the hunt for the primary is unsuccessful, we would then offer a stereotactic biopsy of one of the lesions which we thought would be the most accessible and least likely to lead to complications.

Glial tumours (gliomas)

Glial tumours, or gliomas, are divided into four grades by the WHO classification, the first of these being reserved for the juvenile pilocytic astrocytoma, which is a slow-growing tumour we see in children, and subependymal giant cell astrocytomas, which are intraventricular slow-growing tumours that we infrequently see in adults. Tumours are graded according to their histological characteristics, and four features are searched for: mitosis, nuclear polymorphism, neovascularity, and necrosis. Tumours which have only mitotic features or nuclear polymorphism are usually graded as Grade II, whereas where there is evidence of new blood vessel formation the tumours are usually classed as high-grade, or Grade III gliomas. Tumours where the tissue growth is so rapid that the tissue outstrips its blood supply, and therefore undergoes areas of necrosis, are by definition Grade IV tumours, also called glioblastoma multiforme (GBM). Because glial tumours are made up of brain tissue, they frequently appear as irregular bits of brain on CT scans before the administration of contrast, and in cases of low-grade tumours there is no enhancement with contrast. The one exception to this rule is the juvenile pilocytic astrocytoma, which enhances vividly, although it remains a Grade I tumour. The usual reason for enhancement of a tumour is because of the new blood vessels forming inside the tumour, and enhancement with contrast denotes a high-grade tumour. If there is added necrosis, it then becomes a fairly obvious diagnosis of glioblastoma multiforme. We therefore find that most irregular-looking enhancing tumours are either metastases (since these also have neovascularity) or high-grade gliomas. Both of these tumours carry a grim prognosis and more than 70% of patients with glioblastoma multiforme are dead within 9 months. These malignancies unfortunately are untreatable and palliation is the only option. The decision to offer a debulking procedure usually hinges on the patient's age, general condition and Karnofsky score (a score derived from the patient's ability to function in everyday life – see Chapter 14, Table 14.6). Patients who present at an advanced age with malignant tumours carry the worst prognosis. This is due to the fact that they are medically less fit, and also because these tumours are usually much more aggressive biologically than tumours that present in younger patients. The basis of treatment of these malignant tumours is a debulking procedure without damage to normal brain, followed by radiotherapy. Only a single treatment of radiotherapy can be given to any one patient, and therefore regrowth after radiotherapy leaves only the option of further debulking and chemotherapy. Most patients, as noted before, do not survive very long, but there are a few notable exceptions, and therefore if patients have good Karnofsky scores and wish to have their tumours treated, they should be offered treatment.

Oligodendrogliomas

Another type of primary brain tumour is the oligodendroglioma, which is made up of oligodendrocytes. This is a slow-growing tumour, which enhances irregularly with contrast, just like the malignant tumours, but is usually found in the frontal lobes and may have lots of calcification in it. Because calcium is hyperdense like bone, tumours of this type are usually hyperdense on CT scan before contrast, and are relatively easily diagnosed. They are more benign than the malignant gliomas, and patients have been known to survive a long time with these tumours. Debulking and chemotherapy is usually indicated in the anaplastic variant, with these tumours being very chemo-sensitive.

Non-Hodgkin's B-cell lymphoma

Another tumour which is hyperdense before contrast, but less intensely so, and usually located in a periventricular location, is non-Hodgkin's B cell lymphoma. Because the brain does not have a lymphatic system, all of these are theoretically metastatic tumours, although there is a distinct difference between patients with a known systemic lymphoma and patients in whom the tumour appears to function as a primary brain tumour. These tumours are particularly common in patients with HIV-AIDS. They enhance with contrast quite uniformly. They carry quite a grim prognosis and usually need multi-modal therapy.

Intraventricular tumours

Intraventricular tumours are fairly rare, and the differential diagnosis would be tumours arising from the arachnoid cap cells (meningiomas), from the choroid plexus (papillomas or carcinomas), from the subependymal lining (subependymal giant cell astrocytomas), and from the ependyma (ependymomas). Another benign intraventricular lesion is a colloid cyst, a hyperdense cystic lesion in the third ventricle, which obstructs the foramina of Munro and can lead to sudden death. Midline tumours in the pituitary fossa and pineal region can also invade and extend into the ventricular system because of its close proximity. These are, however, extra-axial tumours.

18

Posterior fossa tumours

In adults, an intra-axial posterior fossa tumour is either a metastatic tumour, a haemangioblastoma, or more infrequently, a glioma. Haemangioblastomas are benign tumours, which consist of a largely cystic component and a small mural module. They can usually be excised quite successfully with surgery. In a small number of cases, a posterior fossa haemangioblastoma can be part of von Hippel Lindau syndrome. This syndrome is typified by the presence of two or more of the following:

- A positive family history of von Hippel Lindau (autosomal dominant inheritance).
- Posterior fossa haemangioblastoma.
- A retinal haemangioma.
- Renal cysts or carcinoma.
- Pancreatic cysts or carcinoma.
- Epididymal cysts.
- A phaeochromocytoma.

A small number of patients also suffer from increased red blood cell production secondary to excess erythropoietin secretion.

Extra-axial tumours

Meningiomas

Meningiomas arise from the arachnoid cap cells in the dura and are mostly benign tumours. They arise from the covering of the brain and cause symptoms and signs by compressing the brain just as an extra-axial collection of subdural or extradural blood would. They have also been called dural warts due to their appearance. These tumours are peripherally located and are diagnosed by the fact that they always have dural attachments. They are frequently very vascular and the distinguishing sign on CT scanning is that they enhance vividly with contrast. Surgery on these lesions can, therefore, frequently be quite tricky, with great blood loss. To try to prevent this they are often embolized preoperatively to reduce their vascularity.

Pituitary region tumours

Brain tumours in the pituitary region are also extra-axial, and the differential diagnosis for tumours in the pituitary region would be pituitary adenoma, metastasis, meningioma, vascular cerebral aneurysm, epidermoid tumours, germ-cell tumours, arachnoid cysts, or craniopharyngiomas.

Pituitary adenomas. Pituitary adenomas are either functional (secreting hormones) or nonfunctional (non-hormone secreting). The more usual hormone-secreting adenomas are prolactinomas, which may be microadenomas (<1 cm), mesoadenomas (1–2 cm), or macroadenomas (>2 cm). There are also cortisol-producing adenomas (usually microadenomas), growth-hormone-producing adenomas, or thyroid-stimulating-hormone-producing adenomas.

Prolactinomas. Prolactinomas cause the clinical picture of galactorrhoea and amenorrhoea in women, and impotence and hypogonadism in men. Cortisol-producing adenomas cause Cushing's disease and growth-hormone-producing adenomas produce acromegaly in adults and gigantism in children.

Craniopharyngiomas. Craniopharyngiomas are benign lesions, which take a long time to grow but cause problems because of compression of the hypothalamus and obstruction of CSF flow. These tumours are thought to arise from remnants of Rathke's cleft, and are classified as adamantomatous or papillary. The adamantomatous type is found in children and is more aggressive; the papillary type is found in adults and is less aggressive. These tumours have an epithelial lining and enlarge slowly by the shedding of this epithelium into the cavity. The resulting keratin and cholesterol crystals cause this tumour to be different on imaging from a macroadenoma. On CT scanning, they usually have multiple areas of calcification and enhance with contrast; on magnetic resonance imaging (MRI), they have a variable appearance but are frequently hyperintense on T1 and T2, indicating not just the fluid content but also fat content due to the cholesterol crystals. Children will usually present with growth retardation, other pituitary deficiencies and visual defects. Adults are more likely to present with visual field defects and pituitary dysfunction.

Aneurysms

Aneurysms can present like tumours with mass effect, and, if they are large, they are visible on CT scanning and enhance with contrast, just as tumours would do. Taking a biopsy from an aneurysm unfortunately leads to drastic consequences and one must take care not to fall into this trap. Angiography is, therefore, a useful investigation if there is any doubt.

Pineal region tumours

Tumours in the pineal region (just posterior to the third ventricle) are either made up of the substance of the pineal gland (pinealomas and pinealoblastomas), or are germ-cell tumours. Pinealomas are tumours with fairly good prognosis. Pinealoblastomas are very aggressive tumours. Germ-cell tumours are either germinomas or teratomas, and they can frequently be diagnosed by doing serum markers for human chorionic gonadotrophin (β-HCG), fetal alkaline phosphatase or alpha-fetoprotein. They are usually extremely radiosensitive and there is also great controversy over whether they should be resected, biopsied, or whether they should undergo radiotherapy without any form of surgery.

Cerebellopontine angle tumours

Tumours in the cerebellopontine angle may be acoustic neuromas (vestibular schwannomas), meningiomas, metastases, arachnoid cysts or epidermoid tumours.

Vestibular schwannomas are nerve sheath tumours arising on the vestibular nerve; they are slow-growing, benign tumours and frequently are associated with neurofibromatosis type 1 (NF1, von Recklinghausen's disease) and neurofibromatosis type 2 (NF2). The gene for NF1 is located on chromosome 17q11.2 and codes for the protein neurofibromin. Although more than half of NF1 cases are due to an inherited autosomal dominant mutation, there is a significant proportion of sporadic new mutations. NF2 is due to inactivation of the schwannomin gene located on chromosome 22q12.2. Clinical manifestions of NF1 include: neurofibromas (commonly on skin); skin abnormalities (café au lait spots); axillary freckling; and Lisch nodules (neurofibromas on the cornea). A small number of these patients also have optic gliomas. Skin abnormalities are less common in NF2 patients, but the presence of bilateral acoustic neuromas is pathognomonic.

Vestibular schwannomas usually present with tinnitus and hearing loss; facial nerve dysfunction is, however, infrequent, even though these tumours usually compress and splay the anterior located seventh nerve during growth. In tumours smaller than 3 cm, radiosurgery can be quite successful. Patients with larger tumours usually need surgery and most surgeons will monitor small tumours for growth before planning surgery.

One controversy surrounding acoustic neuromas relates to whether they should undergo radiosurgery or open surgery. Situations where radio-surgery might be beneficial include:

• Lesions <3 cm

• Where hearing preservation is important

• Medically unfit patients

• Patients who request it.

Surgery is preferred in patients who are medically fit with large lesions, smaller tumours that are growing, or for patients who have indicated that they would prefer surgery.

Another controversy is whether one should aim for a posterior fossa approach, or a translabyrinthine approach. Hearing is usually lost whichever approach is used. However, hearing preservation is normally seen when a posterior fossa approach is undertaken, or when the tumour is very small and a middle fossa approach is undertaken. A middle fossa approach is uncommon in the UK. In the proper hands, these tumours carry a very good prognosis. The main complications are postoperative facial nerve palsies, other cranial nerve damage, and CSF leaks.

Epidermoid tumours

Epidermoid tumours are inclusion tumours and they consist of epithelium. They are enclosed at the time of neural tube folding during embryogenesis and are similar to craniopharyngiomas, in the sense that they slowly enlarge because of epithelial cell desquamation. They are benign tumours but, like the craniopharyngiomas, are impossible to remove totally; luckily, however, they have a very slow growth pattern. Craniopharyngiomas and epidermoid tumours can be treated only with surgery since radiotherapy has little effect on them.

Intracranial vascular disorders

Bleeding into the cranial space frequently has disastrous consequences. Bleeding can either be intraparenchymal, or can occur in the ventricular, subarachnoid, subdural or extradural spaces. The mechanism can either be traumatic or spontaneous. It should also be borne in mind that intracranial vascular abnormalities may present without bleeding, due to their compressing local CNS structures.

Spontaneous bleeds

Cerebral aneurysms

Spontaneous bleeds are due to abnormal vasculature, and in cases of cerebral aneurysms this is due to weakness and out-pouching of the tunica interna and media through deficient external layers of the blood vessels. This is thought to be a flow-related mechanism and is usually found at vessel bifurcations at the site of the greatest flow. Because the blood vessels are located in the subarachnoid space, aneurysms usually lead to subarachnoid bleeds. There is, however, a percentage of aneurysmal bleeds that either also have a parenchymal component or are completely intraparenchymal with no subarachnoid component. Usually there has been a previous leak which has caused some fibrosis between the fundus of the aneurysm and the parenchyma, so that when this ruptures, instead of leaking into the subarachnoid space, it leaks straight into the parenchyma of the brain, presenting like a cerebrovascular accident (CVA) with a deep blood clot in the brain tissue. Aneurysms are classified according to their size, i.e., small (<10 mm), large (>10 mm), giant (>25 mm), or their location, i.e., which blood vessel they arose from (internal carotid, bifurcation, anterior communicating artery, middle cerebral artery, basilar artery, posterior cerebral artery, posterior inferior cerebellar artery, etc).

Making the diagnosis of SAH is critical, and there are two components to it. The first is identifying the blood on a CT scan, and the second is demonstrating the breakdown products of blood by spectroscopy. CT scans are 98% sensitive in the first 12 h after the ictus for detection of SAH, but decline in sensitivity after that to about 70% by day 3. It is, therefore, quite possible to miss the diagnosis if CT scans are used as the only diagnostic modality. If blood enters the CSF, the red cells lyse and oxyhaemoglobin is liberated. This is then converted to billirubin, a process which takes 12 h; this can only happen *in vivo* since the enzyme is found only in the brain itself. CSF in a test tube will therefore produce oxyhaemoglobin secondary to lysis of red blood cells, but not bilirubin because of the absence of the enzyme. The presence of bilirubin can have only one explanation: that there has been blood present in the subarachnoid space for at least 12 h, thus confirming the diagnosis of SAH. This underlies the extreme importance of waiting 12 h before doing the lumbar puncture (LP). If it is done before 12 h it will be negative for bilirubin and may allow blood to be introduced into the subarachnoid space, therefore making any further testing a futile exercise. Doing the LP more than 12 h after the ictus will make the diagnosis successfully in 100% of cases for 2 weeks. The steps involved in making a diagnosis of SAH are summarized in Figure 3.1.

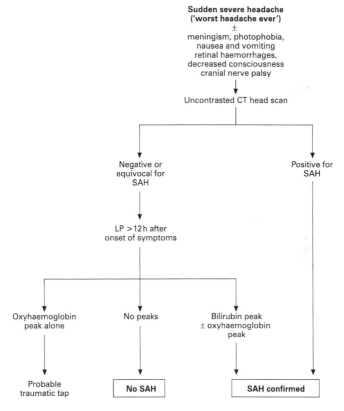

Figure 3.1. Flow chart demonstrating the decision-making process in the diagnosis of subarachnoid haemorrhage.

Arteriovenous malformations

In an AVM there is a short-circuit between the arterial and venous systems without an intervening capillary system; this leads to a shunt. Patients with these conditions may present with a bleed due to the stresses placed on the fragile venous system, with epilepsy secondary to brain irritation, or with a steal phenomenon (where there is cranial dysfunction of certain parts of the brain which are starved of blood supply because of the short circuit). Around 80% of AVMs will have haemorrhaged by the time the patient has reached the age of 50 years, and there is an increased incidence of bleeding during the third and fourth decades. AVMs are classified according to the Spetzler-Martin (SM) grading system, which has a 1–5 grading. Points are given for size, eloquence of brain and the depth of the draining veins. The size is subdivided into lesions smaller than 3 mm, between 3 and 6 mm, and larger than 6 mm. Location depends on whether the lesion is in an eloquent area (motor/speech area, visual cortex, etc.), and the venous draining system depends on whether it drains superficially or into the central deep veins of the brain. A maximum of 3 points will be given for size, and an extra point added for eloquence or deep-draining vein, giving a maximum score of 5. Small AVMs less than 2 mm can be treated with radiotherapy, but these lesions can take several years before they completely obliterate. Lesions larger than 2 mm that are located superficially in non-eloquent brain can be treated surgically. Other lesions can be treated with a combination of endovascular treatment and surgery, or with endovascular treatment alone. SM grades 4 and 5 are not surgically curable in most instances and it may be safer not to treat.

Cavernous angiomas

Cavernous angiomas are bundles of sinusoidal capillaries which have no arterial supply or venous drainage and have a propensity to bleed. Whereas AVMs can be diagnosed with either conventional, CT, or magnetic resonance angiography, these lesions cannot be demonstrated by angiography, and have to be searched for with conventional MRI scanning. They are thought to be surgically treatable if superficial.

Venous angiomas

Venous angiomas are just coils of veins and can be seen as abnormal areas of veins on angiography and usually do not require any treatment. Venous angiomas, AVMs and cavernous angiomas bleed into the parenchyma and should be searched for in patients who are in their first 6 decades and have had spontaneous bleeds.

Strokes

Strokes can be occlusive or haemorrhagic. Occlusive strokes are due to either venous or arterial occlusion and can have secondary haemorrhagic transformation. Haemorrhagic strokes are usually found in the region of the internal capsule and caudate nuclei where the lenticostriate branches of the middle cerebral artery are found. This is usually because of micro-aneurysms forming on these arteries, secondary to hypertension. Cerebellar hypertensive bleeds are also common, and, less frequently, hypertensive bleeds can be seen in other areas in the different lobes of the brain (lobar hypertensive haemorrhage). Strokes usually occur in older people and are in deep inaccessible brain, and therefore are usually not treated with surgery. The exceptions would be patients who have a cerebellar hypertensive bleed, who are deteriorating secondary to hydrocephalus because of obstruction of the fourth ventricle, and in young patients with nondominant hemisphere lobar bleeds which are close to the surface of the brain.

Traumatic bleeds

Trauma can lead to haemorrhage, either because of direct impact or because of the secondary effects of rotation. Very high velocity impact, like being struck by a baseball bat, is dampened quite successfully by the immersion of brain in CSF and leads only to focal damage. This usually manifests as skin lacerations and subepidermal and subgaleal haematomas, or skull fractures which can lead to tears in the arteries on the dura, such as the middle meningeal artery which can, in turn, lead to extradural haematomas. We also sometimes see subdural haematomas following focal impact. Slower impact and rotational movements, like being involved in a car accident or falling down stairs, lead to the brain's being shaken around inside the skull. This leads to diffuse brain injury; in a mild form, it leads to concussion, and in a severe form, it leads to patient's remaining vegetative, secondary to diffuse white matter damage. As the brain gets shaken around, tearing of the axons takes place and, on a microscopic basis, the diagnosis of diffuse axonal injury can be made. There are three grades of diffuse axonal injury (Grade 2 and Grade 3 patients carry a poorer prognosis):

Grade 1. Patients who suffer injury with the appropriate mechanism and have point bleeds through the parenchyma of the brain on CT scanning.

Grade 2. The presence of point bleeds in the parenchyma and point bleeds in the corpus callosum.

Grade 3. Point bleeds in the dorsolateral brainstem.

Patients with acute subdural haematomas usually have a component of diffuse brain injury, and the subdural haematomas usually result from rotational movement and tearing of the bridging veins between the brain and the dura. Patients with extradural haematomas frequently do not have intrinsic brain damage, but become symptomatic because of external compression of the brain, and, if treated promptly, usually carry a good prognosis. In patients with acute subdural haematomas, the bleed is a manifestation of a more serious underlying brain injury, and the response to treatment is variable. In practice, we usually see a mixture of focal and diffuse brain damage. Smaller pin-point contusions are frequently interspersed with larger bleeds in the parenchyma, called haemorrhagic contusions. These are usually found at the tips of the temporal lobes where the brain tissue comes into contact with bone, and also the inferior frontal lobe, as the brain moves over the rough orbital ridges of the cranial floor. Finding subarachnoid and intraventricular blood indicates that there has been a severe diffuse brain injury.

Because subdural haematomas are caused by blood vessel disruption and, in severe cases, parenchymal disruption, it follows that the mechanism of injury leading to diffuse brain injury (and, on a microscopic level, axonal injury) is tailor-made to cause subdural collections. Diffuse brain injury and subdural collections are, therefore, frequently found together, carrying a grim prognosis. Point bleeds may enlarge to become haemorrhagic contusions. Trauma can also lead to intraparenchymal bleeds; these are usually close to the cortex or come to the surface of the brain.

Extradural collections are caused by focal trauma. Due to the fact that the underlying brain is frequently undamaged, they carry a good prognosis if evacuated promptly before brain herniation sets in. Mixed pathology, resulting in both a diffuse injury and a focal injury, is seen, for instance, in cases where a patient's head hits the windscreen during a road traffic accident (RTA), followed by the car rolling and subjecting the patient to rotational movements and diffuse injury. Contact and focal injuries also frequently lead to *coup–contra-coup* type injuries where soft tissue swelling and skull fracture denotes the site of impact clinically and on CT scan, and an intraparenchymal haematoma or haemorrhagic contusion in the opposite part of the brain denotes contact injury which occurred when the accelerating brain came into contact with the skull.

Disorders of CSF flow

CSF is actively produced by the choroid plexus and ependyma and passively absorbed by the arachnoid villi. The ventricular system in the adult contains approximately 150 ml of CSF and approximately 20 ml/h (nearly 0.5 litres per day) is produced. It follows that, if there is no resorption, the intracranial cavity will be rapidly overinflated with CSF. The irreversible consequence of this is death. Overinflation with CSF leads to dilatation of the ventricular system (ventriculomegaly).

Obstructive (noncommunicating) hydrocephalus

Ventriculomegaly due to an obstruction of CSF flow between the ventricles is characterized by some of the ventricles being over inflated whilst the others, being downstream of the obstruction, remain of normal proportion. This type of ventriculomegaly due to an obstruction is called obstructive hydrocephalus or noncommunicating hydrocephalus. Obstructive (noncommunicating) hydrocephalus can be caused by external compression of the ventricular system by bleeds or tumours or by intraventricular obstruction by tumours or bleeds. Obstruction within the body of the lateral ventricles will lead to only a portion of that ventricle being dilated. Obstruction at the foramen of Munroe will cause the whole lateral ventricle to dilate (anterior horns, body, posterior horns, atrium and temporal horns). Obstruction at the level of the third ventricle obstructing both foramina of Munroe will lead to both lateral ventricles becoming dilated, and lesions at the level of the aqueduct will cause dilation of the lateral ventricles as well as the third ventricle, with the fourth ventricle being of normal calibre. In the cases of aqueduct stenosis, the pressure can be relieved by making a small hole in the floor of the third ventricle with an endoscope during a third ventriculostomy. Ventriculoperitoneal shunting is a very successful treatment of obstructive hydrocephalus.

Communicating hydrocephalus

Hydrocephalus can also occur from failure of CSF absorption by the arachnoid villi. The arachnoid villi can be damaged by infection, SAH, high protein states, and increased venous pressure (e.g., sinus thrombosis). Because there is free communication between the ventricles, this type of ventriculomegaly is known as communicating hydrocephalus. Communicating hydrocephalus can frequently be managed by serial lumbar punctures. If the condition does not clear up, shunting may become necessary.

Hydrocephalus is an excellent demonstration of the Monroe–Kelly doctrine which states that, because the cranium is rigid, the three tissues contained (brain, blood and CSF) have an inverse relation to each other, such that an increase in one leads to a decrease or compression of the other two.

Normal pressure hydrocephalus

Normal pressure hydropcephalus is a term used to describe communicating hydrocephalus in the elderly. It is a misnomer, as the intracranial pressure is usually raised intermittently. Young people usually have small ventricles and so diagnosing hydrocephalus is quite easy in them. In older people, it can be quite difficult. As we get older our brain atrophies, and in keeping with the Monroe–Kelly doctrine this creates more space for CSF, since the blood flow, which is the third intracranial component, does not increase. CSF is, therefore, seen to fill the spaces created by the shrinking brain and this translates on a CT scan to large ventricles, or ventriculomegaly, and enlarged sulcal and cisternal spaces. This is a normal state of affairs. When the ventricles enlarge disproportionally to the cisternal and sulcal spaces, this is called ventriculo-sulcal disproportion and points to a high pressure within the ventricular system. The diagnosis is then suggested of communicating hydrocephalus in the setting of relatively normal intracranial pressure, or normal pressure hydrocephalus. The pathology behind this is thought to be a reduced absorption of CSF due to obliteration of subarachnoid spaces and arachnoid villi dysfunction. The key to diagnosis rests on the clinical picture, which consists of Adam's triad of dementia, ataxia and incontinence, as well as the demonstration of a relative increase in CSF pressure of around 20 cm H_2O on LP. The absolute confirmation comes from an improvement in the symptoms (especially gait) following the removal of 30–50 ml of CSF *via* LP. This then confirms that the symptoms of dementia, ataxia and incontinence are not due just to a normal ageing process. It follows, therefore, that if fluid could be permanently drained off *via* a ventriculoperitoneal shunt, a resolution of symptoms might be expected. The principle is that the shunt, having a valve which opens at a certain pressure, would not allow the pressure to rise above that level. The shunt can have either a fixed valve which has a predetermined pressure or a programmable valve which can be adjusted by an external magnet; the second situation allows the valve to be adjusted in the outpatient department to titrate CSF flow, and so obtain the optimum clinical benefit for the patient.

Benign intracranial hypertension

Another type of CSF absorption dysfunction which leads to a rise in intracranial pressure is thought to be caused by increased venous sinus pressure and is called benign intracranial pressure or pseudotumour cerebrii. This is seen predominantly in young, overweight women and is sometimes due to venous sinus thrombosis. There is certainly nothing benign about this intracranial hypertension despite the name. Due to the decreased absorption of CSF there is a general brain swelling and this diffuses down the length of the optic nerve causing venous stasis in the optic nerve and optic nerve swelling. The main complaints are severe high-pressure headaches and peripheral field deficits. There is no ventriculomegaly (hydrocephalus) in these cases and the ventricles are usually slit-like. Once again, the diagnosis is made by demonstrating high pressures in excess of 20 cm H_2O on LP and demonstrating a decrease in symptoms following drainage of 30–50 ml of CSF. Most cases are managed medically with weight loss, diuretics and sometimes steroids. The visual symptoms can sometimes be alleviated by optic nerve fenestrations done by the ophthalmologists. The headaches and the optic symptoms can frequently be improved by CSF diversion by a shunt. Because the ventricles are usually quite small, and therefore difficult to cannulate, these patients usually have a lumboperitoneal shunt put in; this consists of a catheter that runs from the intraspinal space at level L3/4 to the peritoneum, running under the skin of the flank.

Causes of shunt failure

Many patients with hydrocephalus are treated with a shunt, most commonly ventriculoperitoneal, though the distal catheter may drain to a variety of body cavities. Shunts are mechanical devices and so may malfunction due to infection, blockage or mechanical failure.

Blockage due to infection within the first 3 months is usually due to organisms implanted during surgery. *Staphylococcus epidermidis* and *Staphylococcus aureus* are the main culprits with *S. epidermidis* three times more prevalent than *S. aureus*. The predeliction for this organism in shunt infection is due to the fact that it produces a layer of slime under which it hides and which prevents antibiotics and immune cells from entering. That, coupled with the fact that it lives on the skin of both the patient and the theatre staff, makes it the number one suspect. Shunts should be done by senior staff in daylight hours with the minimum staff in theatre, masks should be worn by all present, the shunt should only be handled with instruments and not hands, and contact between the shunt and the patient's skin should be prevented at all times. Shunt infection can present with meningitis-type symptoms (fever, malaise, headache, photophobia, nausea and vomiting), with raised inflammatory markers, or with symptoms of raised intracranial pressure. Patients may have only raised ICP without external signs of sepsis but with elevated inflammatory markers. The only definite proof of shunt infection is a positive gram stain and culture. It is necessary, therefore, to obtain a CSF sample, either by tapping the reservoir of the shunt or during open revisional surgery for blockage. We need continually to drain CSF, and therefore we need a catheter to drain the ventricle. Leaving the shunt in and giving antibiotics alone is one possible method of treatment if the shunt is not blocked. However, this has only a 20–30% chance of success. In the still-functioning shunt, removing the distal end to let it drain into a drainage bag whilst giving antibiotics is another option. The CSF collected in the bag is tested from time to time; when the CSF clears of organisms for a good 24–48 h the old shunt is removed and replaced with a new one. This appears to be a very successful way of treating infection of a patent shunt system. In shunt blockage, the best option is to remove the shunt and use an external ventricular drain (EVD) draining into a drainage bag to allow the CSF to clear (as in the option above, where the functioning shunt was externalized distally). Another option is to replace the infected, blocked shunt straight away with a new one. Many neurosurgeons find this option less desirable, however, as placing a piece of plastic into an environment with an abundance of organisms puts the new the shunt at high risk of being colonized and infected (remember the slime layer of *S. epidermidis*). A further discussion on the management of shunt problems can be found in Chapter 7.

Congenital disorders presenting in adulthood

Aqueduct stenosis

This is an infrequent cause of obstructive hydrocephalus. Aqueduct stenosis due to congenital anatomic abnormality is not as common as aquired aqueductal stenosis due to external compression.

Chiari malformations

Chiari (Arnold–Chiari) malformations are divided into four subtypes: patients with types III or IV usually die shortly following birth, so only types I and II, therefore, will be seen in clinical practice. It is important to note that Chiari malformations are sometimes referred to as hindbrain hernias for reasons that are evident from the following descriptions.

Chiari I

Chiari I is the adult type and usually presents in the 4th decade of life with a mean presentation at 38 years. The deficit is thought to be due to a large foramen magnum, small posterior fossa and possibly perinatal anoxia. The cerebellar tonsils herniate through the foramen magnum and become compressed. On MRI scanning this is seen as tonsils protruding beyond a line drawn from the anterior to the posterior rim of the foramen magnum. Clinically these patients present with cough headaches, myelopathy and tetraspasticity, vertigo, downbeat nystagmus and the symptoms of syringomyelia. The cough headaches are thought to result from CSF being forced past the tonsils into the posterior fossa. This may also be the cause of an associated syringomyelia. In syringomyelia there are cystic spaces within the spinal cord leading to dysfunction of the sensory modalities, especially spinothalamic sensation, as well as motor dysfunction (spastic paresis being the most common abnormality). Treatment consists of an occipital approach and enlarging the bony rim of the foramen magnum as well as incision of the dura, and duraplasty. Some surgeons do not open the dura as they not only feel that doing so may increase the risk of complications, but believe that not doing so does not reduce the success rate of the procedure.

Chiari II

As in Chiari I, the cerebellar tonsils are herniated through the foramen magnum, but in Chiari II the 4th ventricle and medulla have also herniated beyond the line connecting the anterior and posterior rims of the foramen magnum. Chiari II usually presents in infancy with hydrocephalus and respiratory distress (see Chapter 9, on paediatric neurosurgery). It is usually associated with myelomeningocoele.

Intracranial Infection

Introduction of infection into the nervous system can be by several routes. Direct inoculation can occur during penetrating trauma or during surgery (the infected planes can either be extradural, subdural or intraparenchymal, depending on the extent and site of the inoculation). Haematogenous spread may occur from more distant pathology. This is frequently the case in patients with infected granulations on their heart valves, poor dental hygiene, or abscesses at other sites. The usual presentation is that of intracranial abscesses. Direct spread may occur from nearby paraspinal abscesses or infected cranial sinuses. This usually leads to the formation of an extradural or subdural empyema.

Patients with fever accompanied by convulsions should be assumed to have intracranial sepsis until proven otherwise. It is as easy as that. This is a condition with a great morbidity and mortality. Urgent CT scanning with contrast administration is required to demonstrate the infection and, if this is negative, MRI scanning should be considered since this is more sensitive. Aggressive treatment with high dose antibiotics and emergency surgical drainage is indicated. Long-term antibiotics should be administered intravenously for 6 weeks and oral antibiotics continued until all inflammatory markers and imaging have returned to normal. In some cases this may take months. This is especially true for intracranial abscesses since the protective abscess capsule can be resistant to antibiotic penetration. It is important to appreciate that an abscess can take up to 2 weeks to develop a capsule. The earliest stage of intracranial abscess formation consists of a patchy infection of the parenchyma, known as cerebritis.

SPINAL DISORDERS

There is a bewildering variety of pathology that affects the human spine. The main types of spinal pathology in which the neurosurgeon becomes involved include: tumours; degenerative disease; infection; and, more rarely, bleeds. In addition, there are developmental deformities that may require correction. There are various spinal cord syndromes that result from spinal disease, and it will be useful to become familiar with these. These are, therefore, discussed at the end of this section on spinal pathology.

TUMOURS

It is useful to consider the types of malignancy that most commonly occur in the spine according to the various anatomical spaces that they occupy. Extradural tumours are usually metastatic in nature. They are usually centered on the bone of the vertebra (which has a very good blood supply) with intraspinal extradural extension. Intradural tumours are divided into extramedullary and intramedullary tumours. Intradural extramedullary tumours are usually meningiomas or neurofibromas. Intramedullary tumours are either astrocytomas or ependymomas in the majority of cases.

The basis of treating metastatic spinal tumours is, as in the case of brain tumours, palliation. The main aims of surgery would be to decompress the spinal cord in patients with rapidly progressing deficit, and to stabilize the spine in cases of instability. The main treatment for these tumours consists of radiotherapy and this should be commenced as soon as possible once a tissue diagnosis has been obtained (either by open surgical biopsy or needle biopsy). Intradural extramedullary tumours are well suited to surgical resection and are mostly benign. Intramedullary tumours are also treated with surgery, and ependymomas are usually more benign than the astrocytomas. Radiotherapy is also used as adjuvant therapy.

DEGENERATIVE DISEASE

Neural compromise due to compression is usually due to the bony compression of spinal stenosis or to disc degeneration and prolapse. The areas where the stable segments of the spine (the thoracic and sacral spines) join the more mobile segments of the spine (the cervical and lumbar spines) is where the most stress is placed and disc degeneration and prolapse occurs. The most usual segments for this are C6/7, C5/6 and C7/T1 in the cervical spine, and L4/5 and L5/S1 in the lumbar spine. Thoracic disc disease is more unusual. Patients who present with disc prolapse usually do so in the first four decades of their life and there is usually a precipitating event, such as a fall or picking up a heavy object. The disc is composed of a central soft part, the nucleus pulposus, and a tougher outer fibre layer, the annulus fibrosis. Damage to the annular fibres leads to damaged disc material herniating through into the spinal canal. There are various ways in which the separate stages of disc prolapse can be described. In our opinion, the following four terms provide a useful descriptive classification.

1. *Disc bulge:* annular damage with the disc material bulging but still contained by the annular fibres.
2. *Disc protrusion:* the disc fragments protrude through the annular fibres.
3. *Disc extrusion:* the disc material has completely migrated outside the anatomical boundaries of the disc space. On an MRI scan this is seen as a fragment bulging into the spinal canal.
4. *Sequestered fragment:* a piece of disc has broken off and lies loose within the canal.

The single all-encompassing term for the above is *disc prolapse*. The usual initial symptom from disc prolapse is back pain followed by radicular (nerve root) pain. Radicular pain is pain that is caused by nerve root compression and the pain manifests in the dermatome supplied by that specific nerve root.

It is important to understand the anatomy of the spine and the relation of the nerves to the surrounding structures, and to tie that in with the anatomy of the dermatomes. The nerve root of a corresponding segment leaves under the pedicle of the vertebra of that segment. Thus the L5 nerve root leaves under the pedicle of L5 which is opposite the L5/S1 disc space. The nerve root of L5 thus lies quite lateral in the anatomical area opposite the L5/S1 disc space and will be compressed by a disc prolapse which is off the midline in the lateral recess and neural foramen. A disc prolapse in the midline will compress the S1 nerve root on its way to the nerve root foramen under the pedicle of S1. Therefore, at any one given level, a lateral disc will compress the nerve root of that level, whilst a central disc herniation will compress the nerve root of the level below. Compression of a nerve root leads to numbness and paraesthesia, pain and muscle weakness. We can work out from the sensory symptoms and the dermatomes which nerve root is being compressed. The other diagnostic tool is myotome dysfunction: e.g., a central L4/5 (compression of L5 nerve root) disc prolapse will lead to weakness of ankle dorsiflexion and toe dorsiflexion, whereas a L5/S1 disc prolapse (compression of S1 nerve root) will lead to weakness of ankle eversion and plantar flexion with a dropped ankle reflex.

Cervical disc disease causes neck pain, radicular symptoms and myelopathy. Because of the presence of spinal cord in the cervical area (rather than nerve roots as in the lumbar region), central disc herniations will compress the cord and lead to a myelopathy with spasticity in all four limbs. A lateral disc will compress the nerve root and lead to radicular symptoms with pain, numbness and paraesthesia and weakness. A broad central disc can cause both a myelopathy and a radiculopathy, and patients are said to have a radiculomyelopathy. We can once again identify the level according to the dermatomes and myotomes. Spinal stenosis is a disease of general wear and tear and usually occurs from the 5th decade onwards. In the cervical area this leads to slowly progressive myelopathy and sometimes to acute paresis following a sudden extension injury, such as a fall following a slip in the bathroom. The critical diameter of the cervical cord is about 13 mm and compression beyond that leads to symptoms of myelopathy and weakness.

Spinal stenosis in the lumbar area leads to claudication. Unlike arterial claudication, which can occur at rest, neurogenic claudication usually follows walking, and, in severe cases, just standing. The pain is in the calf and is relieved by flexing the hips and standing bent over or sitting down. This leads to less strain on the nerve roots and usually relieves the pain. Spinal claudication is therefore posture related and the pulses are readily palpable, denoting an adequate vascularity. Spinal stenosis is thought to begin with disc degeneration, leading to excess mobility. This is thought to lead, in turn, to facet joint hypertrophy and ligamentum flavum hypertrophy, with resultant auto bony fusion, as the body tries to negate this mobility. Eventually, there is a decrease in spinal canal diameter and the patient becomes symptomatic due to compression of the neural structures.

Spinal stenosis is treated surgically by decompressive laminectomy. Surgery for a disc prolapse is in the form of a discectomy. However, it is important not to forget that conservative management of disc prolapse can be very successful. Discectomies can be *via* a number of approaches, including microdiscectomies (*via* a small bony opening of only a part of the lamina), hemilaminectomies, full laminectomies, or *via* lateral approaches to the exit foramina for laterally placed disc prolapses.

INFECTION

Infection of the spine follows the same basic pathological principles as in the brain, and three mechanisms – metastatic spread, direct extension and direct inoculation – are responsible for infection. Metastatic cancer spreads to the vertebral bodies, whereas metastatic infection spreads to the disc space causing discitis with severe local back pain, pressure tenderness over the affected segment, fever, and raised white cell count and inflammatory markers. Discitis frequently leads to extradural empyema with compression of the thecal sac and the spinal cord contained within the upper spine and the cauda equina contained in the lower part of the lumbar canal. These patients are not only toxic, but also have neurological deficits. Extradural empyema is a feared complication of epidural anaesthesia, and discitis can follow discectomy. Treatment of discitis involves strict bed rest and a long course of IV antibiotics (usually >6 weeks). Extradural empyema requires emergency surgical drainage, followed by bed rest and antibiotics.

SPINAL CORD SYNDROMES

It is helpful to split these syndromes according to whether they occur in the upper or lower parts of the spinal canal.

Syndromes of the upper spinal cord
Anterior spinal cord syndrome
This is due to dysfunction of the cord tissue supplied by the anterior spinal artery and can follow occlusion or damage to this artery, or it is due to anterior compression. It is manifested by muscle weakness below the level of the injury as the motor fibres have an anterior course in the spine. Usually, soft touch (carried anteriorly) and pain and temperature sensation (carried laterally) are also involved. This is an extensive lesion with usually only proprioception (carried posteriorly) intact, and carries a poor prognosis.

Central cord syndrome
This is usually due to hyperextension injury in the elderly where an already critically narrowed diameter of a spinal canal leads to cord compression. The motor fibres in the spinal cord are arranged with the lowest fibres – to the legs – being outermost and the fibres of the arms being innermost. A central cord syndrome therefore damages the inner fibres more than the

outer fibres, leading to arm weakness that is greater than leg weakness. There is usually a variable amount of sensory deficit as well.

Bell's cruciate paralysis

This is seen in victims of trauma who have intact function of their legs but weakness in their arms. This is because the arm fibres cross higher in the spine than do the leg fibres, and a focal injury of the central spinal cord at the point of decussation leads to this phenomenon.

Syndromes of the lower spinal cord

Remember that, in the lower part of the lumbar canal, beyond the conus, there are only nerve roots (cauda equina).

Conus medullaris syndrome

This is due to compression of the conus, which is at L1/2 level. This is the origin of the cauda equina, and compression leads to both spinal cord compression (myelopathy with spastic weakness and sensory deficits) and nerve root compression (radiculopathy with pain, paraesthasia and lower motor neurone flaccid weakness as well as sphincter disturbance).

Cauda equina syndrome

This is frequently seen as a neurosurgical emergency due to sphincter dysfunction. Compression of the roots leads to the usual radicular symptoms of pain, paraesthesia and weakness, but the more sinister component is the compression of the sacral nerve roots that supply perianal, perineal, rectal and bladder sensation as well as sphincter control of both the bladder and the rectum, and erectile function in males. Emergency surgery to remove the compressive element is needed within 24 h of the onset of urinary incontinence/retention or rectal incontinence to save sphincter function. Saddle anaesthesia is usually a warning symptom of pending catastrophe.

PERIPHERAL NERVE DISORDERS

Peripheral nervous system pathology is predominantly the territory of the neurologist. However, there are various peripheral nerve compression syndromes that are amenable to treatment by neurosurgeons.

Compression of the median nerve under the flexor retinaculum leads to pain in the median distribution, as well as to paraesthesia. This is known as carpal tunnel syndrome. Patients frequently awake from sleep with a severely painful hand which improves with elevation. The history is distinctive and tapping over the flexor retinaculum can elicit the symptoms in severe cases (Tinnel's sign), as can holding the wrist fully flexed for >60 s (Phalen's sign). The diagnosis is confirmed with electromyography (EMG) studies, and surgical treatment includes carpal tunnel decompression (see the section on basic surgical procedures).

Ulnar nerve compression can occur in the forearm at the wrist (Guyon's canal) or at the elbow, leading to pain, paraesthesia and paralysis in the ulnar distribution. Surgical release can be quite successful, e.g., ulnar nerve transposition at the elbow.

Peripheral nerve dysfunction may also be caused by peripheral nerve or nerve sheath tumours.

4
Neurosurgical History and Examination

W. Adriaan Liebenberg and Reuben D. Johnson

CONTENTS

INTRODUCTION

Taking a good history and performing a competent neurosurgical examination requires a basic level of knowledge and understanding of the various types of neurosurgical pathology. It is for this reason that this chapter follows the preceding overview of neurosurgical pathology. You should endeavour to use the history and examination to produce a fairly reliable working diagnosis and to localize pathology. Bear in mind non-neurosurgical pathology (e.g., acutely ischaemic legs can mimic a cauda equina lesion), so make sure to enquire about vascular symptoms and feel (and document!) for relevant pulses. The history and examination discussed here are focussed on patients who are alert enough to be on the ward.

HISTORY

This is the most important of all. Listen carefully and allow patients sufficient time to speak. There is no such thing as a 'poor historian' – rather it is a reflection of a lack of skill on our part as history-takers. Have a diagnosis in mind when you have finished, or at least a differential diagnosis; otherwise ask more probing questions to help yourself. Be able to verify which part of the nervous system the pathology is most likely to be located in, and roughly what type of disease process you are expecting. For instance, in the patient who has difficulty walking, it is important to appreciate, and to differentiate between, spinal and cranial pathology, and equally important to distinguish between the different types of pathology – vascular, degenerative, oncological, etc. Be sure to find out, therefore, whether the history is progressive or of sudden onset. You should by now have some appreciation of the significance of different types of headache, e.g., early morning headaches (raised intracranial pressure), sudden onset occipital headache (subarachnoid haemorrhage, SAH), cough- or strain-related occipital headache (hindbrain hernia). Relevant associated symptoms should be inquired about, e.g., fevers, photophobia, alterations in vision, urinary and faecal continence. Be sure to ask about relevant risk factors and associations, e.g., in patients with SAH ask about smoking, family history, polycystic kidney disease.

HISTORY CHECK-LISTS

It may be useful when you start out in neurosurgery to write down a series of check-lists to be covered for different types of patient. Write down the key questions that need to be asked of each patient and perhaps any questions you feel may help in distinguishing between the differential diagnoses. The following are examples of how question check lists can be helpful.

Headaches

Common causes of headache in neurosurgical patients include vascular causes (subarachnoid haemorrhage, AVM), CSF problems (hydrocephalus,

CSF leak), tumours, infection, trauma. Key features in the history will help differentiate between the causes.

1. Onset: sudden (vascular) or gradual (tumour, hydrocephalus, infection).
2. Location, nature, duration, course (episodic or progressive).
3. Associated signs or symptoms. Whilst nausea and vomiting may be nonspecific signs with any cause of raised intracranial pressure, other features, such as swallowing problems, may be associated with Chiari malformations.
4. Exacerbating and/or relieving factors. Whilst hydrocephalus may be associated with worsening headache in the supine position, CSF leak may be associated with increased headache on standing.

Facial pain

The most likely reason that patients with facial pain will be seen in a neurosurgery ward is because of trigeminal neuralgia. The history should be focussed on ascertaining whether or not the pattern of pain fits the criteria for trigeminal neuralgia.

1. Is it paroxysmal (seconds to <2 min)?
2. What is the distribution of the pain (which divisions of the trigeminal)?
3. What is the severity of the pain?
4. Are there any triggers (wind, shaving, eating, brushing teeth)?
5. Are there any associated neurological deficits (there should not be with trigeminal neuralgia)?
6. Has it been relieved by medication (e.g., carbamazepine)?

Spine patients

In all spine patients accurate information needs to be ascertained from the history regarding patterns of pain, motor function (can the patient walk?), sphincter function (bowel and bladder), sensory loss (spinal levels). In patients with back pain be certain to try and ascertain some idea about the aetiology of the pain. Remember that, although back pain is common in degenerative spines it can also be caused by discitis and tumours. In addition, there are certain questions which it is useful to ask for specific cases. For example, in patients with cervical myelopathy it is revealing to ask about function: can the patient do up their buttons/shoe laces?; can they run to catch a bus? Another feature to ask about is shooting pains down the arms and legs (Lehermitte's). In sciatica patients it is important to ascertain whether the pains pass below the knee or to the foot, and whether or not there is any foot drop (foot dragging).

Pituitary patients

It is useful when taking a history from a pituitary patient to think about the symptoms that may arise due to the mass effect of the lesion and those that may arise as a result of endocrine dysfunction. Expansion of a pituitary lesion can cause visual field defects (compression of optic nerve), diplopia/facial pain. Endocrine sequelae will depend upon the type of endocrine disturbance. Female prolactinoma patients may have menstrual irregularities. Panhypopituitary patients may complain of loss of libido, worsening memory, fatigue, and hair loss (often not needing to shave). Acromegalic patients may notice enlargement of their hands when their wedding ring gets tight, or of their feet when their shoes become too small. Cushing's patients may report weight gain, diabetes, mood swings, and joint pains.

Movement disorders

Patients with movement disorders can be challenging for neurosurgical trainees as these patients are predominantly managed by neurologists. However, with the increasing number of functional neurosurgery units these patients are commonly seen on neurosurgery wards. It may be helpful to think about symptoms according to anatomical regions. Ask about basal ganglia region symptoms (tremor, rigidity, bradykinesia, dystonias). For tremor and rigidiy it is important to ascertain which limbs are affected, whether tremors occur at rest or with purposeful movement, and whether there are any precipitating or relieving factors (e.g., alcohol). Ask about walking and whether it is difficult to get going or to stop. Ask whether there are any uncontrolled movements of the face, trunk or limbs (dystonias). For Parkinsonian patients ask about on/off periods and the side effects of medications. Ask patients about cerebellar symptoms(ataxia, nystagmus). Patients may have numerous problems in these complex disorders and so it can be very helpful to determine which symptoms they are most bothered by, and which they would change if they could.

EXAMINATION
THE AWAKE PATIENT

This is by no means a comprehensive and detailed overview of the intricacies of neurological examination. It attempts, however, to give broad guidelines and background that would be useful in everyday practice. Being pleasant and open in your approach helps patients to settle down quickly and be more compliant. It is very important always to have a system. There are several approaches, and the following is a comfortable one. Remember always to introduce yourself and explain to the patient what you are doing.

General observation

Take your time to observe the patient, otherwise important signs such as a Horner's, facial weakness or abnormal movements may be missed. Look for scars, particularly in patients who have had previous neurosurgery. Key areas to check include:

- Behind the ears (cerebellopontine angle surgery);
- The front and back of the neck;
- The arms (neural compression syndrome surgery);
- The vertebral column;
- The chest and abdomen (shunt patients).

In patients with shunts *in situ*, be sure to follow a shunt from the top to the bottom and feel for any breaks in the shunt tubing. Some patients may not recall where their shunt is placed, so do not assume that a shunt is always peritoneal, as it may be placed in the atrium of the heart or the pleural cavity.

General observation is particularly important in pituitary patients. Acromegalic patients may have large hands, coarse features and a large tongue. Cushing's patients may have the classic moon face and acne. Panhypopituitary patients may have smooth skin with little hair.

Mental function and orientation

A quick assessment can be made by asking patients a series of questions about themselves and their surroundings. The questions below constitute the abbreviated mental test score (AMT score) which is given out of 10 (1 point for each question). A common mistake is to refer to this as the mini-mental state examination (MMSE). However, the MMSE takes longer to do, includes drawing tests and is scored out of 30.

1. What is your age?
2. What time is it (to the nearest hour)?
3. Can you remember this address – 42 West Street (recall at end of test)?
4. What year is it?
5. Where are you now (name of hospital)?
6. Can you tell me who these people are or what they do (recognition of two people, e.g., a nurse, a doctor)?
7. What is your date of birth?
8. What year did World War I start?
9. Can you name the present monarch?
10. Can you count backwards from 20 in threes?

More detailed assessment of higher cerebral function should measure orientation, attention, memory (short and long term) and some testing of cerebral lobes: calculation (parietal); abstract thought (frontal); spatial awareness (occipital).

Cranial nerve function

CN I

The olfactory nerve is rarely dysfunctional, except in cases of subfrontal tumours, like meningiomas, or in trauma with an anterior skull-base fracture. Smell function can be tested with a pinch of coffee, each nostril being examined separately whilst pinching the opposite nostril. Intact olfactory function can more conveniently be verified by asking the patient whether they can smell their food.

CN II

We are mostly interested in compression and the dysfunction resulting from it. The optic nerves run in close proximity to the carotid artery and the cavernous sinus, as they extend backwards to the chiasm in front of the lamina terminalis, which is the anterior margin of the 3rd ventricle. From there, they pass around the brain stem to the lateral geniculate body, from where the optic radiations emerge, going to the calcarine cortex in the occipital lobes.

The visual pathways and the defects produced by various lesions in the pathways are summarized in Figure 4.1. Images are transmitted from the retina backwards *via* the optic nerves, with the nasal fibres crossing over and the temporal fibres continuing straight backwards. The lower retinal fibres cross anteriorly (upper temporal visual field) and the upper retinal fibres cross posteriorly in the chiasm (lower temporal field). As the fibres reach the lateral geniculate body, the fibres fan out in an optic radiation, the fibres serving the lower nasal retina (upper temporal field) dipping into the temporal lobe: this part of the optic radiation is known as Meyer's loop. It thus follows that a lesion in the left temporal lobe will cause a deficit in the information carried by the fibres originating on the right nasal retina (upper temporal field). The fibres originating in the left lower temporal retina on the left-hand side also pass through Meyer's loop and a lesion here therefore results in a right-sided upper quadrant homonymous hemianopia. The fibres then reach the calcarine cortex of the occipital lobe where images are recorded, and we become aware of them as the occipital cortex has relays to the visual association areas in the parietal lobes bilaterally. The contralateral relay is much weaker than the ipsilateral relay, and this is the basis for inattention hemianopia. Although a lesion in the right parietal lobe means the patient should not have awareness of an image recorded in the occipital lobe, the patient is nevertheless aware of the image because of contralateral relay to the opposite visual association area. If, however, at the same time, there is an image in the right visual field, which will relay to the left occipital cortex, the ipsilateral input to the left visual association area will obliterate the weaker contralateral input from the right occipital

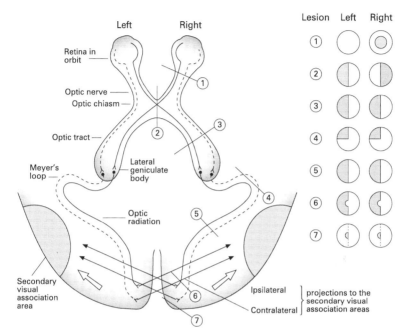

Figure 4.1. Diagrammatic representation of the visual pathways from the retina to the cerebral cortex. The visual deficits shown are due to the lesions indicated: (1) right optic nerve; (2) optic chiasm; (3) right optic tract; (4) right Meyer's loop; (5) right optic radiation; (6) right calcarine cortex; (7) tip of right occipital lobe. Note that the outer part of the visual field may be spared in an early compressive lesion of the optic nerve. The secondary projections to the ipsilateral and contralateral visual association areas are also shown (note that the contralateral projection is much weaker). These are important to understanding the basis of attention hemianopia. If there is a lesion in the right parietal visual association area (serving the left visual field) the contralateral (left parietal) area will allow vision, provided that there is no concomitant input to the left side from the right visual field. This reflects the weakness of the secondary contralateral projections compared to the ipsilateral inputs to the visual association areas. Clinically, attention hemianopia is demonstrated by asking the patient to identify two fingers moving in each side of the visual fields. If the patient can identify fingers moving in one side of the field when they are moved alone but not when fingers in both sides are moved, then they have an attention hemianopia.

area and the patient will no longer see the image in the left visual field (see Figure 4.1). We can demonstrate this in practice by testing visual awareness with a finger placed in the contralateral visual field to where the lesion is, and showing that introducing a finger into the ipsilateral visual field to where the lesion is, causes the patient no longer to see the initial finger.

Understanding the basics of the visual relay helps us to locate a lesion accurately from visual confrontation. This is done by sitting opposite to the patient with your eyes at the same level as theirs; you then ask the patient to block off their right eye with their right hand while you block off your left eye with your left hand. Then, starting on the left-hand side, you bring your finger (or a red pin) in from the periphery and you note the position in which the patient detects your finger (or the pin). The reason for using a red pin is that an inability to see red is the first deficiency that appears with optic nerve compression. This procedure, known as the confrontation test, is done in superior, lateral, inferior and medial peripheries of one eye and then repeated with the other eye, with the patient similarly occluding their eye. This easily demonstrates any field deficit that might be present. Remember to document the visual fields as the patient would see them. The presence of intact vision and full visual fields indicates a free flow of information along the optic nerves. Any deficit, therefore, is a sign of compression or obstruction to the flow of this information.

The four typical lesions that we find are:

- A lesion of a single optic nerve before it reaches the chiasm: this will result in loss of vision in a single eye Therefore, a compression, or loss of function, of the left optic nerve will result in left eye blindness.
- A lesion compressing the chiasm: this will initially compress only the nasal fibres which cross over, because the temporal fibres, which do not cross over, are more laterally situated. This lesion will lead to a loss of vision in both temporal visual fields.
- A lesion in the temporal lobe: this will, as described previously, lead to a contralateral upper quadrant homonymous hemianopia.
- A lesion in the parietal or occipital cortex: this will lead to a contralateral homonymous hemianopia of both the upper and the lower quadrants.

Assessing visual acuity is also an intrinsic part of testing the function of the optic nerve, although people can have near complete obliteration of their optic field and still have intact visual acuity. Visual acuity is tested with an eye chart at a distance of 6 m. The vision is documented as a fraction of 1; a value of 1 indicates normal vision, i.e., an ability to read the 6 m line with the chart placed at 6 m (denoting the ability to see the same size letters as a person with normal vision would be able to see at 6 m). The patient with the worst recordable vision would be one who could see at 6 m only letters of a size that a person with normal vision would be able to see at 60 m; therefore it is recorded as one tenth of normal vision, or 6/60.

The third and last step of testing the optic nerve is by doing fundoscopy. It is, perhaps, the case that never have more lies been told in medicine than in the reporting of fundoscopic results. There is frequently general confusion about fundoscopy, and the skill to diagnose papilloedema comes only with repeated examinations of different normal fundi. The term papilloedema means bilateral disc swelling and should be reserved for that. It is best to note down whether optic disc swelling is left-sided or right-sided. Papilloedema takes 10–14 days to develop, and is thus unlikely to be present in acute neurosurgical pathology. It is therefore important to realize that lumbar puncture in a patient with intracranial pathology might be hazardous, even though the fundoscopy is normal. There are four very easy-to-remember stages in the development of papilloedema.

Stage 1. The back pressure in the optic nerve leads to decreased ability of the veins to drain, and therefore there is an increase in venous calibre and tortuosity. It is also possible, with experience, to see a decreased venous pulsation.

Stage 2. Because of the swelling, the optic disc changes from its normal pale colour to pink, and starts to swell, causing the vessels that usually plunge into the disc to stop abruptly at its margins.

Stage 3. The disc margins have now become indistinct and blurred.

Stage 4. The disc now is elevated, pink and swollen, and it is quite common to see haemorrhages around the veins.

Fundoscopy is useful, therefore, for detecting papilloedema that is usually present in cases of long-standing tumours or hydrocephalus, but it is also useful for detecting haemorrhages. In SAH we do see – albeit infrequently – retinal and vitreous haemorrhages (Terson's syndrome) and subhyaloid haemorrhages (bleeding beneath the subarachnoid membrane).

CN III, IV, VI

Examination of the oculomotor nerve has two components. The third cranial nerve works together as a team with the second cranial nerve to constrict the pupil, and works together with the fourth and sixth cranial nerves to move the eye around in the orbit. A light-stimulated impulse travels back in the optic nerve to reach the lateral geniculate body; then, in the brain stem at the level of the superior colliculus, fibres are given off bilaterally to the Edinger-Westphal nuclei. From the Edinger-Westphal nuclei a parasympathetic pathway passes through the brainstem, quite close by an area called the conversion centre, into the third cranial nerves of both sides. Both the Edinger-Westphal nuclei and both oculomotor nerves are thus activated by input from a single side, and we therefore have a bilateral, consensual reaction to a unilateral input (see Figure 4.2). As the impulse travels down the oculomotor nerves, it reaches the ciliary ganglion from where the short ciliary nerves serve the sphincter pupillae to cause a pupillary constriction. The fibres of the oculomotor nerve that mediate sphincter constriction lie on the surface of the nerve on the dorsal aspect and are, therefore, usually involved quite early on in compression of the third nerve. Pupil constriction is therefore a parasympathetic function, mediated by the third nerve following activation of a parasympathetic nucleus by the second cranial nerve. Damage to the afferent pathway (retina, optic nerve, chiasm and optic tract) leads to a pupillary response known as the Marcus Gunn pupil. This is elicited by swinging a flashlight in a pendulum motion between the two pupils. As the light falls on the unaffected eye, both pupils will constrict fully because of the afferent input on both Edinger-Westphal nuclei. As the light falls onto the affected eye, the affected pupil will, instead of constricting, slightly dilate because of the decrease of afferent input due to afferent pathway damage. Efferent pathway lesions lead to a loss of constriction and therefore to dilatation of the pupil served by the oculomotor nerve, which denotes dysfunction caused either by intrinsic mechanisms or by extrinsic compression. The fact that the pupillo-constrictor fibres lie superficially on the third nerve is an important distinguishing factor between medical dysfunction of the third nerve and a surgical (compressive) lesion.

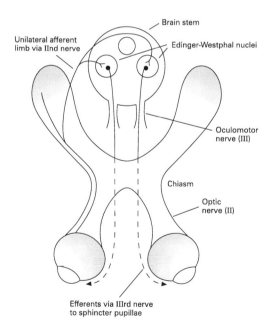

Figure 4.2. Diagrammatic representation of the afferent and efferent limbs of the pupillary reflex. Note that the afferent limb conveys impulses from a single eye to both Edinger-Westphal nuclei. This is the basis of the consensual light reflex where light shone into one eye causes bilateral pupillary constriction.

Third nerve dysfunction where there is involvement of the pupil is usually compressive. The third nerve also carries some sympathetic fibres which innervate the superior and inferior tarsus muscles of Muller which assist eye opening. The first component of a third nerve compression is therefore dilatation of the pupil, and the second is ptosis.

Pupillary dilatation is brought about by sympathetic activity, which is initiated in the hypothalamus and then descends down into the spinal cord to the level of T1. At the level of T1, the white rami of the nerve roots of C8 and T1 pass to the cervical sympathetic ganglion and from here sympathetic nerves enter the cranial cavity on the surface of the carotid artery, and are delivered to the pupil *via* a branch of the ophthalmic nerve. Dysfunction of this system leads to ptosis (because of decreased supply to the tarsus muscles), myosis (loss of mydriasis) and anhydrosis (loss of sweating) – the so-called Horner's syndrome.

The second main function of the third cranial nerve is movement of the eyeball, in conjunction with the fourth and sixth cranial nerves. The third cranial nerve supplies all the muscles of the eyeball, except for the superior oblique and lateral rectus muscles: this can be remembered easily using the formula $(LR_6SO_4)3$. A patient with a full third nerve palsy will, as we have discussed before, have a dilatation of the pupil, as well as a ptosis. They will also have a pupil which is looking downwards and outwards. This is because of the unopposed pull of the lateral rectus and superior oblique muscles. The lateral rectus muscle causes the eyeball to look towards the outside, and the superior oblique muscle, which hooks around a trochlea, causes the eye to look inferiorly. It follows that lateral rectus palsy causes an inability of the affected eye to look laterally. It is difficult (and quite rare) to find an isolated fourth nerve palsy: when it does occur, it usually presents with diplopia on looking outward and downward because of superior oblique dysfunction. This can best be conceptualized by recalling that the superior oblique pulls the eye down and medially, whilst the inferior rectus pulls the eye down and laterally. In a patient with a fourth cranial nerve palsy, downward gaze results in the unopposed action of the inferior rectus pulling the affected eye down and out. Downward gaze, therefore, precipitates or worsens diplopia.

CN V

The three branches of the trigeminal nerve traverse the cranial cavity in three separate places: the mandibular nerve enters through the foramen ovale; the maxillary nerve enters through the foramen rotundum; and the ophthalmic division through the superior orbital fissure. The trigeminal nerve is mostly sensory and supplies sensation to the whole face. The mandibular nerve carries the motor part and this supplies the muscles of mastication. Examination of the trigeminal nerve primarily tests the sensation of the first, second and third division, as well as the corneal reflex (which is part of the first division). Power of muscles of mastication, as well as the jaw jerk, which are part of the evaluation of the trigeminal nerve, are of lesser clinical significance.

It is important to recall that the third, fourth, and sixth cranial nerves, as well as the first division of the trigeminal nerve, run through the cavernous sinus and can be compromised by lesions there. Patients with intracavernous aneurysms, tumours, or arteriovenous fistulae, frequently have palsies of the third, fourth and sixth cranial nerves, and of the first division of the trigeminal nerve on the ipsilateral side.

CN VII

The facial nerve is almost purely motor, and supplies all the muscles involved in facial expression. It also has a sensory component to the external auditory canal and conveys taste from the anterior two thirds of the tongue *via* the chorda tympani. Clinical evaluation of the seventh cranial nerve hinges on the understanding that there are two separate components to facial nerve function: the first is the supranuclear innervation of the muscles of facial expression, and the second is mainly concerned with reflex eye closure and does not have a cortical component. Both eyes will shut if there is any danger to either individual eye, and therefore there is dual innervation of both sides of the forehead. This leads to the finding of intact upper face function in patients who have had a hemispheric incident, such as a stroke.

The fifth, seventh and eighth cranial nerves are located in a space between the pons of the brain stem, the cerebellum, and the cranial base, in an area called the cerebellopontine angle.

CN VIII

The vestibulocochlear nerve really consists of two nerves, with the cochlear nerve relaying hearing from the cochlea, and the vestibular nerve relaying information from the apparatus of balance (the semicircular canals and otolith organs). Acute events, such as trauma and infection, cause decreased hearing as well as balance problems. Chronic compression leads to a decrease in hearing, though balance remains intact due to compensation by the contralateral vestibular function. Hearing can be crudely tested by rubbing your fingers together at the side of the patient's ear and determining whether or not the patient can hear the movement. Webber and Rinne testing can be extremely useful to distinguish between conductive and sensorineural deafness. If more information is needed about hearing function, a patient should be referred to an audiologist.

CN IX, X, XI

The ninth, tenth and eleventh cranial nerves are usually tested together. The reason for this is anatomical. These three nerves share the same motor nucleus, the nucleus ambiguus, in the medulla (although the accessory also has a spinal nucleus) and they all exit the skull by the same route (through the jugular foramen). This close anatomical association within the confines of the skull means that it is unusual for centrally located pathology to produce isolated lesions of these cranial nerves.

The glossopharyngeal nerve (IX) is the main afferent path of the gag reflex, supplies some sensation around the external auditory canal, and conveys taste from the posterior third of the tongue. The only clinically significant aspect is the afferent part of the gag reflex. The vagus nerve (X) also helps to convey sensation from the ear but is the main afferent pathway for the gag reflex. The vagus nerve is also motor to most of the muscles of the palate. Testing the ninth and tenth cranial nerves thus consists of testing the gag reflex, which demonstrates an intact afferent pathway (ninth cranial nerve) and efferent pathway (tenth cranial nerve) and also testing palatal function by asking a patient to open their mouth and say 'aah'. If there is a palsy, the muscles that are intact on the unaffected side will pull the palate in that direction and therefore demonstrate the palsy.

The spinal accessory nerve (XI) originates in a nucleus in the spinal cord, leaves the spinal cord through cervical branches, and then goes on to supply the sternocleidomastoid and trapezius muscles on the ipsilateral side. This nerve is unusual in that the higher control is not crossed and a right-sided lesion will therefore lead to a right-sided nerve dysfunction. The function of the eleventh nerve is tested by asking the patient to lift the ipsilateral shoulder up against resistance to test power in the trapezius muscle: the patient is then asked to turn his head away from the side being tested whilst pressure is applied to the head while the patient is looking in the contralateral direction, and the sternocleidomastoid muscle is palpated to check for a good muscle action and bulk. A right sternocleidomastoid and right eleventh nerve function is therefore tested by asking the patient to look towards the left against resistance and palpating the muscle on the right-hand side.

CN XII

The hypoglossal nerve (XII) supplies the motor fibres of the tongue and is tested by asking the patient to open their mouth and let the tongue lie loosely in the mouth. Fasciculations are noted at this point, and the patient is then asked to stick his tongue out and move it from side to side. If there is a palsy, the stronger and intact side will push the tongue over towards the weak side.

Cranial nerve testing

It is extremely important to develop a quick and efficient manner of testing the cranial nerves. Usually the first cranial nerve is not tested, except when there is a clinical suspicion; the second cranial nerve is tested by doing acuity visual confrontation fields and fundoscopy; the third, fourth and sixth cranial nerves are tested together by checking the movements of the eye; the fifth cranial nerve is checked by noting the sensation in the face; the seventh cranial nerve is tested by asking the patient to move their face in a grimace, to whistle, and to wrinkle their forehead; the eighth cranial nerve is tested by rubbing your fingers together close to the patient's ear; and the lower cranial nerves are testing by examining the gag reflex, looking at palatal function, checking shoulder and neck movements, and finally by looking at movements of the tongue. If practised, this can be done quickly and in sequence within a few minutes.

After noting down the history and asking a few pointed questions to ascertain the patient's mental function, and when the cranial nerves are fully tested, it is time to move on to the rest of the neurological examination.

Motor system

As we know, motor function is controlled contralaterally in the cerebral hemisphere, and there can be dysfunction anywhere from the motor cortex, corona radiata, internal capsule, the decussation in the medulla, to the spinal cord and peripheral nerves. These are the so-called pyramidal pathways. Motor function is also dependent on the extrapyramidal system, and upon the modulation supplied by the cerebellum. Table 4.1 summarizes myotomes and dermatomes. Even minor dysfunction can be demonstrated by forcing a patient to rely on both the pyramidal system (intact power) and extrapyramidal system (positional feedback and proprioception). This can be done by asking a patient to hold their arms outstretched in front of them and asking them to make a piano-playing movement in the air. Alternatively, you can ask them to close their eyes and stand with their arms outstretched, palms facing up. Inability to do piano-playing movements, or a drift towards the inside (pronator drift), indicates mild weakness. This is useful for testing patients who have cranial dysfunction. Power is noted on a scale of 1–5, with 5 being normal power, 4 being mildly reduced power, 3 indicating anti-gravity power, 2 indicating movement which is not able to defy gravity, and 1 indicating a flicker. The Medical Research Council (MRC) scale is summarized in Chapter 14 (Table 14.5), which deals with scoring systems in neurosurgery.

The pyramidal system

Trying to decide the location of the dysfunction causing a power deficit can be confusing, but if we stick to a few simple rules it should be fairly obvious. If there is abnormal power, there has to be a dysfunction at some point between the brain and the muscle. In neurosurgery, we do not usually get to deal with muscle abnormalities, and will therefore ignore those. Lesions of the brain pathways or the spinal cord will cause weakness, but will also decrease the higher modulation of reflex activity in the spinal cord. This will cause patients to have overactive reflexes and therefore to appear spastic.

Table 4.1. Summary of myotomes, dermatomes and root values of common reflexes.

Nerve root	Myotome (muscles supplied)	Action	Reflex	Dermatome
C5	Deltoid Biceps	Shoulder abduction Elbow flexion	Biceps jerk	Lateral forearm
C6	Biceps Brachioradialis	Elbow flexion Elbow flexion	Biceps jerk Brachio-radialis jerk	Thumb
C7	Triceps	Elbow extension	Triceps jerk	Middle finger
C8	Flexors digitorum	Finger flexion	–	Little finger
T1	Intrinsic muscles of the hand	Finger abduction and adduction	–	Medial forearm
L1	Hip flexors	Hip flexion	–	Anterior thigh & inguinal area
L2	Hip flexors	Hip flexion	–	Anterior thigh
L3	Quadriceps	Knee extension	Knee jerk	Anterior thigh
L4	Quadriceps	Knee extension	Knee jerk	Anteriormedial thigh
	Tibialis anterior	Ankle dorsiflexion and foot inversion	–	–
L5	Extensor hallucis longus	Big toe extension	–	Lateral leg
S1	Ankle	Plantar flexion	Ankle jerk	Posterior lower leg and lateral side of foot
S2	Ankle	Plantar flexion		

It is important to realize that the lower part of the lumbar spine does not contain spinal cord, but only the cauda equina, and so only lesions above the level of L1/2 will lead to spasticity; a lesion from L3 downwards cannot lead to spasticity. Above L3, the rule that governs the level of dysfunction is different. At the level of the lesion you may find lower motor neurone signs, and therefore weakness without spasticity (decreased reflex), whilst at the level below that you will find weakness with increased reflexes and spasticity. Thus, a cord lesion at C5 will lead to decreased power in the biceps and reduction in the brachioradialis reflex, but spastic reflexes in the fingers and in the lower limbs.

The basis for finding the origin of weakness is the absence or presence or spasticity and the level of that spasticity. For instance, a patient with compression in the thoracic cord will have spastic legs, but normal tone and reflexes in the arms; a patient with compression of the brain or the cervical cord will have both spastic arms and legs. Patients with lumbar disc disease can never be spastic due to their disc. A patient with both facial weakness and a hemiparesis obviously has a cranial dysfunction and needs a computerized tomography (CT) scan of his brain.

Reflexes should be noted as absent, present with reinforcement, present, increased, increased with nonsustained clonus, or increased with clonus.

Extrapyramidal system

The cerebellum is the main modulator of movement, and integrates proprioceptive feedback from all over the body to modify and change motor signals to our muscles. As a general rule, lesions of the cerebellar vermis will lead to truncal ataxia and an inability to stay upright whilst sitting in bed. Hemispheric cerebellar lesions tend to cause ipsilateral limb ataxia. A left cerebellar lesion thus causes ataxia in the left arm and left leg.

A patient with cerebellar disease will usually be hypotonic on the side of the lesion, reflexes will be decreased, and nystagmus is common. Limb ataxia in the upper limbs can be elicited by asking a patient to touch their nose and then to touch your finger which is held about 60 cm or so away from the patient's nose; the movement is then repeated rapidly to and fro. The patient will frequently not be able to touch your finger, and will point past it. There will also be a shaky and unsteady movement of the hand. It is also not possible for the patient to keep their hands outstretched and do piano playing movements (this will already have been picked up in the screening test for motor dysfunction). The lower limbs can be tested for ataxia by asking the patient to run the heel of one foot up and down the shin of the other leg, starting at the knee and returning to it. This will usually be a very shaky and uncoordinated movement if there is ataxia present. The final test to confirm the ataxia is to ask the patient to do rapid and alternating movements, such as tapping his foot on the floor or tapping the back of one hand with the other hand as fast as he can. An inability to do this is termed dysdiadochokinesis.

Evaluation of gait is an often neglected but important part of neurological examination. Patients with severe lower back and radicular pain will have an antalgic type of gait where they put less pressure on the affected side. In patients with cerebellar disease, there is a general unsteadiness due to limb ataxia. In patients with a CVA, there is usually fixed flexion of the upper limb and a straight, outstretched leg with plantar flexed foot, which causes them to walk by circumducting the affected leg (swinging the stiff, outstretched leg out and around before placing it down). Patients who are myelopathic have a stiff and spastic gait and frequently shuffle along.

It is, therefore, quite obvious that a lot can be learned from observing a patient's gait. Romberg's test depends on our need for at least two out of three senses (proprioception, middle ear, vision) to be able to stand unaided. Therefore, closing the eyes will cause patients to fall over backwards or forwards if they have either middle ear pathology or decreased proprioception. As can be imagined, this is not a very specific test, and has little clinical value.

Sensory system

When testing sensation, you basically have to test four modalities: light touch, pain, temperature and joint position sense.

Light touch is tested by lightly touching the patient's skin, either with your finger tips or with cotton wool, down the whole length of the body and comparing results between each side of the body.

Pain sensation is tested with pin-prick and this is usually quite successful in delineating sensory level. It is important to compare normal with abnormal and also to compare the two sides of the body. If you think that a patient has a sensory lesion at the T4 level, it is useful to compare sensation in the face with sensation on the trunk; sensation on the face would probably be normal. Be careful not to fall into the 'C4–T4 trap': these dermatomes are very close on the trunk and it is possible to misdiagnose a C4 lesion as a T4 lesion. We then also have to compare left to right. It is usually unnecessary also to test temperature sensation, since the two modalities, pain and temperature, are closely related physiologically (fibres for both modalities run together in the spinothalamic tracts).

Two-point discrimination is reliable only when tested on the fingertips where discrimination of 3–5 mm should be sensed by a normal patient. Joint position sense should be tested in both hands and both feet, and is quite a reliable indicator of abnormal function of the sensory cortex. There is no specific clinical significance in testing vibration sense.

When testing sensation, we really want either to indicate a level at which sensation changes or ends, or to show a hemispherically-located decrease in recorded sensation, when comparing the two sides. Sensation testing is an aid in localizing pathology and is discussed further in the chapter on spinal disease.

THE COMATOSE PATIENT

Competent assessment of the comatose patient requires accurate assessment of the Glasgow Coma Scale (GCS) score and searching for focal deficits by evaluating pupillary responses and motor function.

Glasgow Coma Scale

The GCS is an excellent tool. Unfortunately, there are too many people who do not fully understand it and seem frightened to use it. Being awake does not equate to a GCS of 15/15, and being difficult to rouse does not mean that the patient is confused. The GCS score is a very biological measurement; it is not a measure of a patient's alertness, so much as of their ability to defend and look after themself. This can be seen when the three components of the GCS are considered in turn.

The motor response

This is prognostically the most valuable part of the GCS. A full mark is 6/6 and the worst mark is 1/6.

> 6/6 being able to follow commands which need a rather sophisticated train of events in the nervous system;
>
> 5/6 aware of, and being able to localize, a painful stimulus (pain) in order to defend oneself (called purposeful flexion or localizing to pain);
>
> 4/6 aware of, and flexing to, but unable to find, the threatening stimulus (reported as non-purposeful flexion);
>
> 3/6 decortication, when the arms are spasmodically fully flexed next to the body (this can be thought of as an action that has no reliance on the cognition of the cortex – decortication);
>
> 2/6 decerebration, when the arms are spasmodically extended on either side of the body, the legs also are spastic and extended (think of a stage of spinal reflex that does not rely on the cerebrum at all – decerebration); this and the previous stage are called posturing, and have a grim prognosis;
>
> 1/6 no motor response.

Speech

A full mark is 5/5. This can sometimes be misleading, as a lesion in the speech area might be small but sufficient to cause a person to lose speech, and thus lead to a score of only 1/5 in the speech component, thereby dropping the total GCS total score to 11/15.

> 5/5 fully orientated with regard to place, time and person (orientation);
>
> 4/5 confused speech without full orientation (confusion);
>
> 3/5 words;
>
> 2/5 sounds;
>
> 1/5 no sounds.

Eye opening

A full mark would be 4/4 and the lowest mark 1/4. Being able to see a threat is crucial to an organism's ability to defend itself.

> 4/4 spontaneously has eyes open;
> 3/4 will open eyes to speech or sound and is aware of surroundings;
> 2/4 so unresponsive that only a painful stimulus is enough to make the patient aware of a threat; is unaware of surroundings;
> 1/4 no stimulus is enough to make the patient open his/her eyes.

Total score

The total GCS score is 15. The lowest GCS is 3/15 and this is true in patients who are fully sedated, those who are only functioning on their brainstem or those who have even lost this primal function and who are thus brain dead. See Chapter 8 on NICU management to see how to test for brainstem function.

Focal deficits

Pupillary function

Pupillary dilatation is a symptom of herniation and increased ICP and it is an important warning sign. This is tested as one of the brainstem reflexes.

Motor function

It is important to establish whether there is a hemiparesis (weakness) or hemiplegia (no function). A comatose or confused patient's examination is usually restricted to the GCS, pupillary response, and presence or absence of a paresis.

5
Interpretation of CT Head Scans
Reuben D. Johnson

CONTENTS

Paraventricular tumours
Temporal lobe tumours
Infection (cerebritis and abscess)
Cortical injury
Diffuse axonal injury
Cortical contusions
Infarction
Some common cysts
Arachnoid cyst
Colloid cyst

INTRODUCTION

Identifying neurosurgical abnormalities on computerized tomography (CT) head scans need be no more difficult than interpreting a chest X–ray. Similar principles apply.

Confirm the patient details and date of the scan. This also helps you to put the scan up correctly since to read the patients details you have to have the scan the right way up and not back-to-front. Identify whether the scan is with or without contrast. Work through the scan in an ordered and systematic fashion. If there is an obvious abnormality, describe all its features, i.e., site, shape, density and homogeneity, and whether or not it enhances. Ensure that you go back and check all your review areas to make sure you don't miss anything. To be able to do all these things, you need to have a system of working through the scan, and to know how to identify the gross anatomical structures on a CT scan so that you can localize the lesion. You will also need to know the terms that are used to describe cranial CT lesions. It will be useful to have a simple mnemonic to ensure you have checked everything.

CRANIAL ANATOMY ON CT SCAN

You need to able to identify the following areas: spaces (ventricular system, cisterns); parenchyma (lobes of hemispheres, cerebellum, brainstem, basal ganglia); dural folds (tentorium, falx); sinuses (sagittal sinus). Figure 5.1 shows the main features of a normal axial CT head scan.

DESCRIBING LESIONS

Describing lesions is very important. You should be able to describe a scan over the phone to a senior colleague. It is essential to use a system and terms that everyone is familiar with and understands. The following features of a lesion should be covered when describing them on scans.

- *Site*: anatomy (see above); is the lesion intrinsic (within the parenchyma) or extrinsic (arising outwith the parenchyma, but may be pushing into it)?

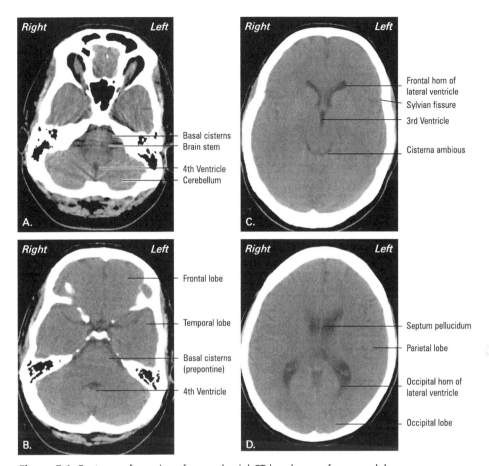

Figure 5.1. Features of a series of normal axial CT head scans from caudal (A) to rostral (D). The key features that should be identifiable on a CT head scan are annotated. Note that the location of the right and left side of the patient reflects the radiological convention of looking at scans from a caudal viewpoint.

- *Shape*: diffuse or well-circumscribed; smooth or irregular edge.
- *Density*: hyperdense (whiter than brain), hypodense (darker than brain), or isodense (same density as brain).
- *Homogeneity*: homogeneous or inhomogeneous density.
- *Enhancement*: enhancing (regularly, irregularly or ring-enhancing) or non-enhancing; the significance of enhancement is that it indicates that the blood–brain barrier has been breached, or that there is neovascularity.
- *Associated features*: e.g., surrounding oedema, dural origin, calcification.

A SYSTEM OF REVIEW

Start at the bottom of the head and work up through the axial slices.

CSF SPACES

Ventricular system

The ventricular system comprises the 4th ventricle, the aqueduct, the 3rd ventricle, and the lateral ventricles. The aim here is to identify hydrocephalus and, if it is present, to determine whether it is communicating or obstructive. Note in particular the temporal horns (see Figures 5.10, 5.12, 5.13, 5.20 and 5.22). These are not normally visible in younger people and their presence indicates that there is hydrocephalus. Once hydrocephalus has been identified, see whether there is any obvious level of obstruction. For example, if the 4th ventricle is of normal size but the ventricles above (3rd and lateral) are dilated then there must be obstruction at the level of the aqueduct. See Figure 5.13 for a good example of obstructive hydrocephalus due to blood in the 4th ventricle and Figure 5.22 for an example of hydrocephalus secondary to obstruction at the level of the 3rd ventricle.

Basal cisterns

Reviewing the basal cisterns is particularly important as it can help in determining whether or not intervention is required. For example, if an elderly man with a small chronic subdural haematoma has no midline shift and his basal cisterns are widely open, then he may not require intervention as he has room to compensate for the mass effect of the haematoma. On the other hand, if the basal cisterns are completely obliterated in a diffuse head injury then it may be that intervention will not alter the outcome as the patient has already coned. The basal cisterns also communicate with the subarachnoid space and are therefore one of the commonest sites in which to identify subarachnoid blood – see the features of subarachnoid haemorrhage (SAH), below.

SYMMETRY OF BRAIN SUBSTANCE AND TISSUES

Work up from the foramen magnum through the cerebellum, basal ganglia and internal/external capsule to the hemispheres. Look for any symmetry, as any asymmetry indicates that something is wrong somewhere. If there is shift to one side, examine the contralateral side carefully for any space-occupying lesions. Look in particular at the sulci and sylvian fissures. They may be effaced if there is a compressive lesion. It is useful to look at the skull and the extracranial tissues as any asymmetry due to fractures or scalp swelling can give clues to the presence of intracranial lesions. If anything abnormal is seen, try to identify which part of the brain it is in. Does the location of the lesion conform to the history? A useful tip is that if you can see the falx in the midline, then you are above the tentorium.

CONSISTENCY OF SCAN AND HISTORY

It is essential to confirm that the scan is consistent with the history. For example, a patient with a history of a gradual-onset, right-sided weakness and a scan showing a small, right-sided, acute, basal ganglia bleed does not add up. In this case it would be necessary to look for left-sided pathology, such as infarct or subdural haematoma, or it might be necessary to consider spinal pathology. Also, a scan might look horrendous but the patient might actually be better clinically. In this case, ensure that you have the correct patient's scans and check the date of the scans. Consider carefully the sequence of events. For example, consider a patient who fell off their bike and has subarachnoid blood on the scan. Did they have a spontaneous bleed from an aneurysm and then fall off their bike, or were they knocked off by a car, in which case they may have had a traumatic bleed?

A CHECK-LIST MNEMONIC

The following mnemonic (CT SCAN) provides a useful check-list to ensure that you have not missed anything.

C	CSF flow: ventricular system
T	Tissues: symmetry of intracranial, cranial and extracranial tissues
S	Sulci and sylvian fissures
C	Cisterns
A	Abnormal blood: look for SAH, epidural haemorrhage (EDH), subdural haemorrhage (SDH)
N	Never forget the history! Is the scan consistent with the history?

CT FEATURES OF COMMON NEUROSURGICAL CONDITIONS

To formulate a differential diagnosis you need to know the features typical of common neurosurgical conditions. These conditions have characteristic patterns in terms of site, shape, density, homogeneity, enhancement, and any additional features. It was pointed out earlier that, in very broad terms, neurosurgical pathology can be divided into haemorrhage and tumours. It is useful, therefore, to consider typical CT features of common conditions under these headings. In addition, we will consider CT features of other neurosurgical conditions, namely abscesses, diffuse head injury, common cysts, and infarction.

HAEMORRHAGE

It is useful to remember the different appearances of extravasated blood on CT scans. Acute blood (<72 h) is hyperdense (white), subacute blood (72 h to 1 week) is isodense, and chronic blood (>1 week) is hypodense.

61

Traumatic bleeds

Extradural haematoma (see Figures 5.2 and 5.3)

- Between skull and brain.
- Biconvex (inner convexity pushing into brain) due to the fact that the dura is being stripped away from the bone.
- Hyperdense.

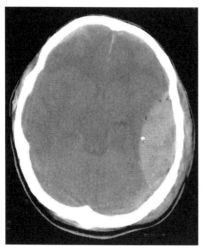 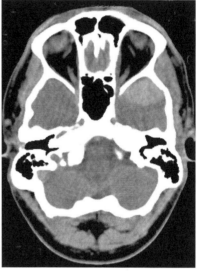

Figure 5.2. Axial CT head scan showing a large, left-sided, parietofrontal extradural haematoma. Note that the haematoma is biconvex and hyperdense. This haematoma is probably due to rupture of the left middle meningeal artery. There are also some hyperdense areas at the frontal poles that may represent contusions from a contra-coup injury. The presence of extracranial soft-tissue swelling on the left side is further evidence that the blow is likely to have been to the left side of the head.

Figure 5.3. Axial CT head scan showing a left-sided temporal haematoma. Note the classic crescentic shape and hyperdense appearance.

Subdural haematoma (see Figures 5.4–5.9)

- Between skull and brain.
- Crescentic (follows contour of brain).
- Hyperdense (acute), isodense (subacute), or hypodense (chronic).
- Loculation and membranes may be visible in chronic subdural haematomas (CSDH).

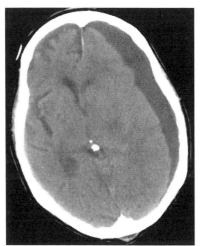 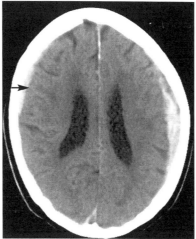

Figure 5.4. Axial CT head scan showing a large, left-sided, chronic subdural haematoma covering the convexity of the whole hemisphere. There is significant midline shift (>1cm) with distortion of the ventricular system. The haematoma is crescentic and hypodense. Note that the sulci over the left hemisphere have been effaced. In smaller haematomas this may be the only sign indicating the presence of subdural blood, especially if the blood is subacute and isodense (see Figure 5.6)

Figure 5.5. Axial CT head scan showing a left-sided, frontoparietal, acute subdural haematoma. The haematoma is crescentic and hyperdense. Note that there is also some acute subdural blood on the right side (arrow).

Figure 5.6. Axial CT scan showing a left-sided, frontoparietal, subdural haematoma (crescentic and hyperdense). Note that there are also some hyperdense areas in the right hemisphere with some associated scatter effect. This is usually seen with radio-opaque foreign material. There are also a couple of hypodense areas within the parenchyma suggesting the presence of intracranial air. Swollen parenchyma is also contributing to the shift to the right side Unfortunately, this patient was shot at close range through the head with a low calibre weapon. The foreign bodies in the right hemisphere are the remnant of the bullet and/or fragments of bone.

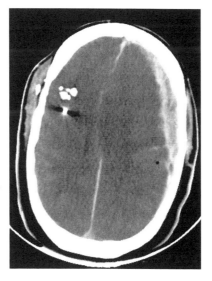

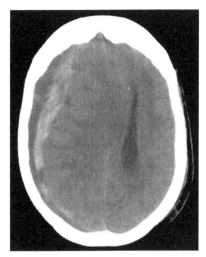 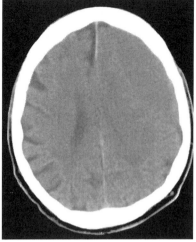

Figure 5.7. Axial CT head scan showing a right-sided, acute-on-chronic, subdural haematoma covering most of the right hemisphere. Note the crescentic shape and the mixture of hypodense and hyperdense areas indicating, respectively, old and new blood.

Figure 5.8. Axial CT head scan showing a large, subacute, left-sided, subdural haematoma. The haematoma is beginning to turn hypodense. However, the clear asymmetry seen in the scan is more evident because of the absence of obvious sulci in the left hemisphere.

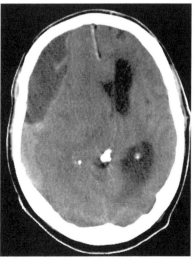

Figure 5.9. Axial CT head scan showing a large, right-sided, chronic, subdural haematoma with massive midline shift. Note that there is a horizontal level demarcating the upper hypodense area from a lower hyperdense area. It is possible that the hyperdense area represents a further acute bleed separated by membranes from the chronic component. However, it is more likely that this is simply sedimentation of an old bleed.

Spontaneous bleeds

Subarachnoid haemorrhage (see Figures 5.10–5.14)

- Subarachnoid space
  - Basal cisterns: circle of Willis aneurysms.
  - Sylvian fissure: internal carotid, posterior communicating artery (Pcomm), or middle cerebral artery (MCA) aneurysms.
  - Interhemispheric fissure and anterior flame-shaped intra parenchymal haemorrhage: anterior communicating artery (Acomm) aneurysm (the most common aneurysm).
- Diffuse streaks following surface of brain.
- Hyperintense – but after 1 week may not be visible due to dissipation by CSF flow. (CT scans are 98% sensitive in the first 12 h for SAH, but sensitivity declines to 70% by day 3).

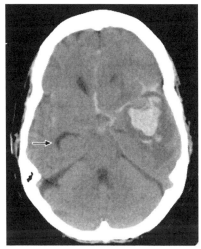 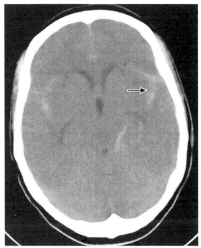

Figure 5.10. Axial CT head scan showing the presence of acute subarachnoid blood. There is also a large left temporal intraparenchymal haematoma (hyperdense). Interestingly, the middle cerebral artery aneurysm responsible for this bleed can be seen silhouetted against this haematoma. The hypodense area around the haematoma reflects the swelling in the surrounding parenchyma. The other noteworthy abnormality is the enlarged right temporal horn (arrow) indicating the presence of moderate hydrocephalus.

Figure 5.11. Axial CT head scan showing the presence of subarachnoid blood (hyperdense). Note in particular the presence of blood in the left sylvian fissure (arrow).

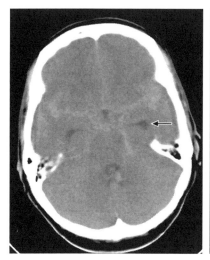
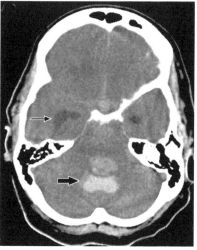

Figure 5.12. Axial CT head scan showing diffuse subarachnoid blood (hyperdense). Note that the temporal horns are slightly enlarged, indicating the presence of hydrocephalus (arrow indicates left temporal horn).

Figure 5.13. Axial CT head scan showing the presence of subarachnoid blood and a large collection of blood in the 4th ventricle (thick arrow). This obstruction of the 4th ventricle is causing hydrocephalus, as evidenced by the enlarged temporal horns on this scan (thin arrow).

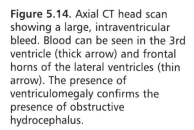

Figure 5.14. Axial CT head scan showing a large, intraventricular bleed. Blood can be seen in the 3rd ventricle (thick arrow) and frontal horns of the lateral ventricles (thin arrow). The presence of ventriculomegaly confirms the presence of obstructive hydrocephalus.

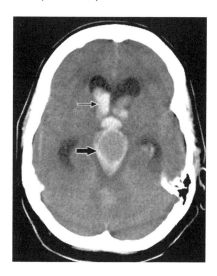

Hypertensive bleeds

- Most commonly basal ganglia and cerebellum, but can be a lobar intraparenchymal cerebral bleed.
- Vary in shape.
- Hyperdense in acute phase.
- Hypodense area may surround clot due to oedema.
- Usually elderly hypertensive patient, but not exclusively so.

AVM

- Similar features to hypertensive bleed but more cortical location and more likely to occur in normotensive younger patients.
- Frequently have an underlying 'salt and pepper' appearance with the mass of underlying vessels faintly visible on an uncontrasted scan and vividly visible following the administration of contrast.

TUMOURS

Metastases (see Figure 5.15)

- Intraparenchymal (intrinsic) and may be multiple.
- Well-circumscribed.
- Mixed density.
- Inhomogeneous.
- Enhancing: either inhomogeneously or ring-enhancing and can have central necrotic areas.

Gliomas

Low-grade (see Figure 5.16)

- Intraparenchymal (intrinsic).
- Regular shape but poorly defined edges.
- Hypo- or isodense.
- Homogeneous.
- Non-enhancing (except for juvenile pilocytic astrocytoma).

High grade (see Figure 5.17)

- Intraparenchymal (intrinsic).
- Irregular and may be diffuse.
- Mixed density.
- Inhomogeneous.
- Strongly enhancing (in an inhomogeneous fashion) with central necrosis in the highest grade – glioblastoma multiforme (GBM).

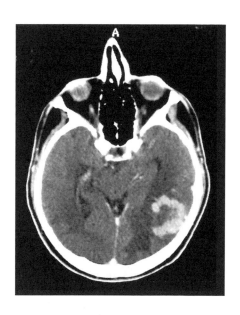

Figure 5.15. Axial CT head scan with contrast, showing a metastasis in the left parietal lobe. Note that the lesion is well-circumscribed, enhancing, and of mixed density. There is probably some central necrosis.

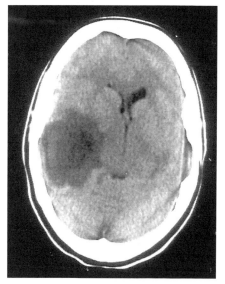

Figure 5.16. Axial CT head scan of a large, low grade glioma of the right parietal lobe. The lesion is hypodense and virtually homogeneous.

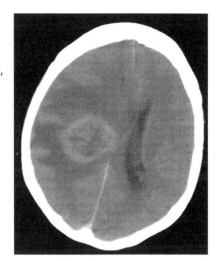

Figure 5.17. Axial CT head scan with contrast, showing a large, right-sided, enhancing, parietal space-occupying lesion with surrounding oedema (hypodense area) and midline shift. The centre of the lesion is inhomogeneous. This is a high grade glioma with a necrotic centre.

Meningiomas (see Figure 5.18)
- Extrinsic – although appearing parenchymal they will always have a dural origin.
- Well-circumscribed smooth or lobular.
- Hyperdense.
- Homogeneous.
- Enhance homogeneously (they light up like a light bulb).
- Skull changes – associated with skull erosion and thought to be a malignant feature. Other meningiomas are associated with hyperostosis, much like fibrous dysplasia.

Oligodendrogliomas (see Figure 5.19)
- Commonly in the frontal and temporal lobes.
- Calcification is almost invariably present.
- Inhomogeneous appearance.
- Inhomogeneous enhancement.

Primary CNS lymphomas (PCNSL)
- Periventricular intraparenchymal (intrinsic).
- Irregular.
- Hyperdense with surrounding hypodensity (oedema).
- Homogeneous.
- Enhance homogeneously.
- Disappear with steroids ('ghost tumours').

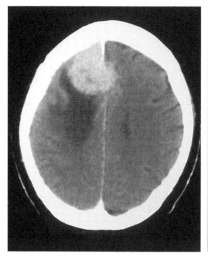

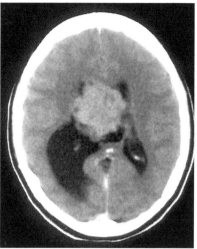

Figure 5.18. Axial CT head scan with contrast, showing a right frontal meningioma. The lesion is enhancing and homogeneous with a dural attachment.

Figure 5.19. Axial CT head scan with contrast, showing an inhomogeneous, intraventricular oligodendroglioma.

Figure 5.20. Axial CT head scan with contrast, showing a ring-enhancing, cystic, space-occupying lesion in the posterior fossa (cerebellum). Note the effacement of the 4th ventricle and the presence of obstructive hydrocephalus as evidenced by distended temporal horns. This is a haemangioblastoma.

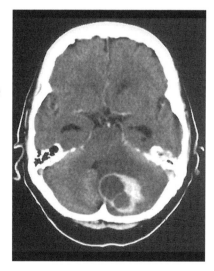

Haemangioblastomas (see Figure 5.20)
• Posterior fossa.
• Regular, well-circumscribed cystic.
• Hypodense but with isodense mural nodule.
• Mural nodule may enhance and become more clear.

Medulloblastomas
• Children.
• Posterior fossa, midline.
• Regular, well-circumscribed.
• Isodense.
• Homogeneous.
• Enhance homogeneously.

Ependymomas
• Mostly in children in the posterior fossa; also in adults and can appear anywhere in the brain.
• In the posterior fossa they usually arise from the foramina of Luschka and Magendie.
• Usually enhance uniformly.

Cerebellar gliomas
• Usually in children, and form the main differential diagnosis of posterior fossa tumours along with ependymomas and medulloblastomas.
• The same imaging characteristics are true as in the cerebral gliomas and they are usually not midline tumours.

Primitive neuroectodermal tumours (PNET)
• Found in the cerebrum in children.
• Have the same characteristics as medulloblastomas.

TUMOURS BY INTRACRANIAL LOCATION

It is extremely helpful to have some appreciation of how the intracranial location of the tumour can help determine what type of tumour it is. In adults, for example, a posterior fossa lesion or parenchymal lesion is most likely to be a metastasis, but a haemangioblastoma should be considered if the lesion is cystic with a mural nodule. In children, posterior fossa lesions are much more likely to be primary brain tumours such as medulloblastomas and pilocytic astrocytomas. Some of the locations which help in the identification of tumour types are listed below.

Intraventricular tumours
• Ependymomas.
• Subependymoma is the only non-enhancing intraventricular tumour.

- Neurocytoma (lobulated, adjacent to septum pellucidum or foramen ovale, hyperdense on CT).
- Pineal tumours.
- Choroid plexus tumours (prominent enhancement): most common in IVth ventricle in adults, but more common in lateral ventricle in children.
- Meningiomas (prominent enhancement).

Paraventricular Tumours

- Subependymal giant cell astrocytoma (SEGA): associated with tuberous sclerosis (cortical tubers, subependymal nodules along lateral ventricles, benign foci of dysmyelination in deep white matter); often arise from the caudate; hypo/isodense on CT.
- PCNSL (see above).
- 75% in contact with ependyma/meninges hence 'pseudomeningioma pattern' (but no calcfications and usually multiple).
- 'Ghost tumour' as may disappear radiologically with steroids.

Temporal lobe tumours

- Dysembryoplastic neuroectodermal tumours (DNET): variable density with variable enhancement.
- Ganglioglioma: cystic; calcified with isodense mural nodules; rarely enhance; rarely associated with oedema; clinical picture is often a child with a seizure.
- Pleomorphic xanthoastrocytoma (PXA): cystic; discrete mural enhancing nodule; presentation in teenage years/early twenties.

INFECTION (CEREBRITIS AND ABSCESS) (See Figure 5.21)

- Encapsulated abscess takes 2 weeks to develop from cerebritis.
- Cerebritis: normal scan or poorly defined hypodense area (may enhance).
- Abscess: well-defined rounded hypo/isodense lesion which 'ring-enhances' with contrast, with the capsule tending to be thinner on the side of the ventricle, and the side of the convexity being thicker.

CORTICAL INJURY

Diffuse axonal injury

- In acute stages, CT may be normal.
- Hyperdense spots (pettechial haemorrhages) in white matter – see the description of the three grades in the pathology section (p. 25).

Cortical contusions

- Patchy areas of hypodensity with sporadic hyperdense spots (pettechial haemorrhages) in acute phase.
- Later, more hyperdense areas develop as bleeding continues and there

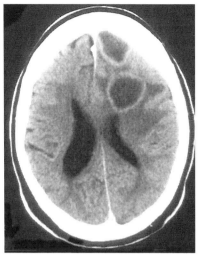 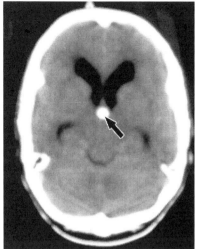

Figure 5.21. Axial CT scan with contrast, of two cerebral abscesses located in the left frontal lobe. The lesions are hypodense and ring-enhance with contrast.

Figure 5.22. Axial CT scan showing a hyperdense colloid cyst in the anterior 3rd ventricle obstructing the foramen of Munro (arrow). Obstructive hydro-cephalus is confirmed by the presence of distended anterior and temporal horns.

is more associated hypodense oedema and mass effect; these lesions develop into haemorrhagic contusions, particularly between days 5 and 7, with maximal swelling and re-bleeding occurring then.
• Temporal lobe and frontal lobes most commonly affected.

INFARCTION
• Normal scan in acute phase.
• Later, areas of low density develop and shape will depend on cause of infarction, e.g., wedge-shaped infarct with MCA occlusion but more diffuse areas with infarction after vasospasm associated with SAH.

SOME COMMON CYSTS
Arachnoid cyst
• Well-defined, hypodense extra-axial lesions (same density as CSF).
• Frequently found in the area of the pituitary fossa and cerebellopontine angle, but can be found anywhere.

Colloid cyst (see Figure 5.22)
• Small, round, hyperdense midline lesion in the anterior part of the 3rd ventricle.

6
Overview of Neurosurgical Investigation and Monitoring
Timothy Lawrence and W. Adriaan Liebenberg

CONTENTS

INTRODUCTION

Some of the major advances in neurosurgery in the second half of the last century have resulted from developments in imaging techniques. There are numerous investigations utilized in order to aid diagnosis and facilitate localization of surgical anatomy. It is therefore paramount that the junior trainee has a basic understanding of these modalities. A brief overview follows of some of the more important investigations you will come across.

COMPUTERIZED TOMOGRAPHY (CT)

The development of computerized tomography nearly 40 years ago revolutionized investigation and diagnosis in neurosurgery. It has now become the standard form of imaging and one which the junior trainee needs to be very comfortable and familiar with. Multiple rotating beams of X-rays pass through tissue. The degree of absorption of each beam is measured by a circular array of detectors. Standard CT allows for 3–5 mm slices; however, a helical CT will allow for finer slices of 1–2 mm and for faster scanning times. Manipulation of the different window settings allows better examination of tissue of varying density. Neurosurgeons are often interested in bony windows and soft tissue windows, allowing for identification of fractures, bony abnormalities, intracranial masses, blood, ventricular shape and size and so on. Contrast administration helps provide additional information about abnormalities picked up on plain scan, such as tumours, vascular abnormalities and infection.

MAGNETIC RESONANCE IMAGING (MRI)

The detailed physics behind magnetic resonance imaging is complicated. Essentially, a magnetic field aligns the spin of molecules within tissue. Hydrogen protons are then displaced by the electromagnetic impulse. As the magnetic field is switched off the tissues return to a resting state. Different tissues return to a resting state at different speeds. By changing pulses of magnetism directed at these molecules returning to their resting state, different image types can be generated. There are two times noted at the bottom of the scan: the first is the time to relaxation (TR), and the second the time to echo (TE). The type of scan sequence is determined by these. There are certain sequences that allow us to visualize clearly certain tissue types.

T1 SEQUENCES

These are sequences that show water (and therefore CSF) as black. They are very good for demonstrating contrast enhancement. T1 images should be compared with T1 sequences with contrast administration (gadolinium – a paramagnetic substance) to highlight areas that enhance. T1 sequences are usually used to identify cranial pathology, and it is common to have axial, sagittal and coronal cuts. Hyperintense lesions before contrast administration can only be fat, blood (acute stage) or melanin. Bone is hypointense, as is calcification. Brain tumours usually return less intense signals and are therefore hypointense (compare with hypodensity of CT scans). They usually have variable enhancement, with contrast becoming more hyperintense (compare hyperdensity of CT scans). The difference in nomenclature between CT and MRI scans is due to the fact that CTs function by the penetration of X-rays through tissues and we therefore talk about density. MRI scan works on the principle of the intensity of the returned signal of molecules in flux, and hence we refer to it as intensity.

T2 SEQUENCES

In T2 sequences the CSF is white and tumours are usually white as well, reflecting the presence of fluid from cystic and necrotic areas as well as from neovascularization. These sequences are particularly useful when looking at spinal pathology since the white CSF makes a good contrast and backdrop to any pathology. Tumours or disc herniations can usually be seen to displace the normal white areas. Cranially, T2 sequences tend to overestimate the size of tumours, as the lesion seen is the tumour plus the surrounding oedema. A variation is the fluid-attenuated inversion recovery (FLAIR) sequence, which demonstrates only abnormal body water and not the normal anatomical CSF collections.

DIFFUSION WEIGHTED IMAGING

Diffusion weighted imaging (DWI) MRI has been increasingly used in recent years. In simple terms, DWI MRI reflects the rate of water diffusion, i.e., DWI is sensitive to Brownian motion of water molecules and calculates the apparent diffusion coefficient (ADC). As a general rule, restricted diffusion is represented by density opposite to that of CSF; e.g., if CSF is black then areas of restricted diffusion will be white. The presence of restricted diffusion on DWI MRI is useful for differentiating between epidermoids and arachnoid cysts, and can be useful in helping to differentiate between a tumour and an abscess.

MAGNETIC RESONANCE ANGIOGRAPHY

Magnetic resonance angiography (MRA) is an excellent noninvasive tool, as is CT angiography (CTA). Both these modalities are noninvasive and are approaching the sensitivity and specificity of the gold standard, conventional digital subtraction angiography.

ANGIOGRAPHY

Conventional digital subtraction angiography is the gold standard for the detection of vascular abnormalities. New advances have been the ability to treat these abnormalities endovascularly and, potentially, to treat complications of subarachnoid haemorrhage (SAH), such as vasospasm. There is a small but definite risk attached to this procedure; therefore it is not used as a routine screening test but only in cases where there is good reason to suspect underlying vascular abnormalities. You should know the basic anatomy on an angiogram and what to look out for in order to be able to diagnose an AVM or aneurysm. There are usually several views done and they are marked in the top corner usually as LICA (left internal carotid artery), RICA (right internal carotid artery) and posterior circulation. There are anteroposterior and lateral views for LICA, RICA, and posterior circulation. See Figures 6.1, 6.2, 6.3 and 6.4 for examples of standard angiogram views.

Make sure that you can read the patient's name and that you have the two LICAs and two RICAs as well as the two posterior circulation sets together. There will also be an oblique or spin view of the LICA and RICA: ignore them for now.

It is important to practise looking at the different arteries in the different views.

The internal carotid passes through the petrous bone and has several

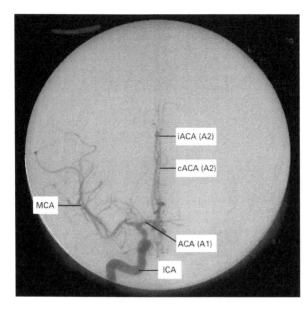

Figure 6.1. Right internal carotid angiogram sequence (postero-anterior view). The vessels are annotated as follows: middle cerebral artery, MCA; internal carotid artery, ICA; anterior cerebral artery A1 segment, ACA (A1); ipsilateral anterior cerebral artery A2 segment, iACA (A2); and contralateral anterior cerebral artery A2 segment, cACA (A2).

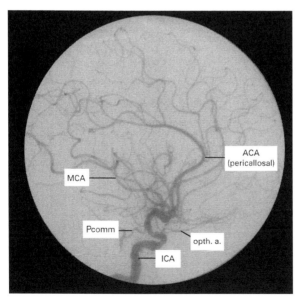

Figure 6.2. Right internal carotid angiogram sequence (lateral view). The vessels are annotated as follows: internal carotid artery, ICA; ophthalmic artery, ophth. a.; posterior communicating artery, Pcomm; middle cerebral artery, MCA; anterior cerebral artery, ACA.

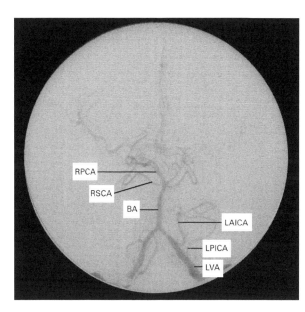

Figure 6.3.
Left vertebral artery angiogram sequence (anterior view). The vessels are annotated as follows: left vertebral artery, LVA; left posterior inferior cerebellar artery, LPICA; left anterior inferior cerebellar artery, LAICA; basilar artery, BA; right superior cerebellar artery, RSCA; right posterior cerebral artery, RPCA. Note that all these are paired, bilateral vessels, apart from the single midline basilar artery.

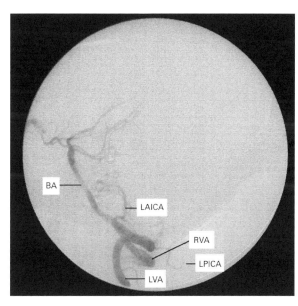

Figure 6.4.
Left vertebral artery angiogram sequence (lateral view). The vessels are annotated as follows: left vertebral artery, LVA; right vertebral artery, RVA; basilar artery, BA; left posterior inferior cerebellar artery, LPICA; left anterior inferior cerebellar artery, LAICA.

twists and turns before passing through the cavernous sinus and exiting through the foramen lacerum into the cranial space. It then has an ophthalmic segment, communicating segment, and a choroidal segment, before it divides into the middle cerebral artery (MCA) and anterior cerebral artery (ACA). The names of these segments are directly derived from the branches that leave the carotid.

The ophthalmic artery runs in an anterior direction and is the first branch seen. This is followed by the posterior communicating artery (Pcomm) slightly higher up, which joins the posterior cerebral artery. The Pcomm is usually slightly larger than the ophthalmic artery, but sometimes it is much larger and this is then called a fetal Pcomm. In the fetus, the posterior circulation is fed by the anterior circulation *via* the Pcomm, and only later in fetal development is the posterior circulation fed by the vertebral arteries and the basilar artery. If this state persists, the Pcomm is hypertrophied and important in the supply of the posterior cerebral territory (occipital lobes).

The next artery is the anterior choroidal artery which is usually within 4 mm of the bifurcation of the carotid and also extends posteriorly. Aneurysms are flow-related phenomena and thus are usually seen at the origin of these arteries rather than distally. Therefore, if you carefully follow the carotid up to the bifurcation, looking at the origins of the opthalmic, posterior communicating, and anterior choroidal arteries, you will not miss aneurysms (looking like round or irregular outpouchings) on these arteries. Do this for both the left and the right sides.

On the lateral views there are two areas to look at now. One is the very busy area where the branches of the MCA are coming directly at us and are quite bundled together on the image, and the other is the area of the ACA, which curves anteriorly and around the corpus callosum, and allows easy identification of the branches as they are seen on their lateral aspect. The ACA has a pre-communicating segment, a communicating segment and a post-communicating segment. The pre-communicating segment is short and extends from the origin of the ACA to the anterior communicating artery (Acomm) which connects the two ACAs. Most aneurysms are found around the Acomm as this is where the most turbulent flow occurs as the arteries change direction. Distal to the communicating segment there are several branches: the frontopolar, callosomarginal, and pericallosal arteries. It is unusual for aneurysms to occur in these branches.

On the anteroposterior view, the MCA artery can be visualized properly and it has two bifurcations where aneurysms usually form: one proximal and the other more distal. This view will also demonstrate which ACA is the dominant artery and whether it flows across to the other ACA *via* the Acomm. This is important, since we usually approach an Acomm aneurysm from the nondominant hemisphere.

The posterior circulation should be filled by both vertebral arteries during angiography, and an anteroposterior view and a lateral view are used to demonstrate aneurysms. Identifying AVMs can take some experience. Angiography is a dynamic process and there will be several images of the same view on one film. This is to demonstrate the filling of the arteries; the last images are the venous phase and start to show up the veins into which the arteries drain. Seeing a vein earlier than expected would mean a shortcut between the arterial and venous system and therefore an AVM. A blush of arteries and veins together can be quite easily seen, and this also denotes an AVM. It is sometimes necessary to demonstrate not only the two internal carotid arteries (ICAs) and two vertebral arteries (four-vessel cerebral angiography) but also the two external carotid arteries (six-vessel cerebral angiography) when there is a suspicion that the arteries supplying the dura contribute to an AVM.

INTRACRANIAL PRESSURE (ICP) MONITORING

Intracranial pressure can be measured from three anatomically distinct locations: subdural, intraparenchymal, and intraventricular. Subdural sensors are the most frequently used and the least sensitive, but carry the lowest risk of infection. Placing the sensor into the parenchyma increases the sensitivity and accuracy of the measurement but increases the risk of infection. Intraventricular monitoring *via* an extra ventricular drain (EVD) is the most reliable and allows the option of draining CSF off when there is an increase in ICP. However this carries the greatest risk of infection. The sensors are attached to a monitor and the pressures are recorded continuously. CSF pressures differ from person to person but a normal pressure is considered to be between 10 and 20 mmHg. Pressure of more than 20 mmHg usually warrants treatment. Looking at the pressure waves on the monitor also provides important information.

Sustained rises in ICP are thought to correlate with secondary brain damage and are therefore an important indicator of deterioration and consequently of the need for intervention. If patients are awake, then clinical examination is used to gauge damage. This is not possible when the patient is asleep, and ICP monitoring therefore provides vital information about progressive intracranial injury. In cases where there are short transient increases in ICP the clinical effect is usually not severe. If there is a continuous increase or a plateau in ICP, it becomes important to treat, as these are usually malignant increases. By measuring the ICP and mean arterial pressure (MAP) we are able to calculate cerebral perfusion pressure (CPP).

$$CPP = MAP - ICP$$

This allows manipulation of blood pressure in order to optimize cerebral perfusion. Pressure monitoring is most commonly used in traumatic brain injury but some centres also use it in other intracranial pathology such as SAH. See the section in Chapter 10 on basic procedures for the insertion of an ICP bolt.

DUPLEX DOPPLER

This is a velocity measurement of blood flow, and is used to provide evidence of vasospasm (arterial narrowing causing a focal ischaemic neurological deficit following SAH). The MCA is usually targeted through the thin squamous temporal bone, but the Doppler technician can also target other intracranial arteries. If the blood flow exceeds 200 ml/s in the MCA, it is indicative of vasospasm. In the awake patient, clinical deterioration is usually the hallmark of vasospasm but duplex Doppler can diagnose vasospasm in the awake and comatose/sedated patient. It is therefore a valuable tool in the treatment of SAH patients.

JUGULAR VENOUS OXYGEN MONITORING

Continuously monitoring the amount of oxygen in the venous blood as it returns from the brain can help to tell us what the oxygenation of the brain parenchyma is like, and this procedure is used in some centres. The aim is to stop the oxygenation from dropping below 60% by manipulating the blood pressure and ventilation requirements. Few units use it routinely.

PERFUSION CT SCANNING

Perfusion CT scans are ordinary CT scans where contrast is administered and a software package calculates the perfusion in the different areas of the brain according to the flow of contrast through it. Other perfusion scans use the administration of xenon gas to calculate blood flow; these can demonstrate regional hypoperfusion states and allow us to modify our therapy.

POSITRON EMISSION TOMOGRAPHY

Only a very few centres have positron emission tomography (PET) as it requires a cyclotron. PET scans are functional scans which can detect radioactive isotopes administered to patients. Oxygen uptake and glucose delivery can demonstrate biological activity and, for instance, differentiate between a tumour or post-radiation necrosis, a distinction which is notoriously difficult to make by other means.

MR SPECTROSCOPY

MR spectroscopy (MRS) can be useful for differentiating between inflammatory conditions, metabolic diseases, tumours, radiation necrososis, and abscesses. MRS provides information about the chemical composition of a lesion. For example N-acetyl aspartate (NAA) is a neuronal marker which is usually decreased in pathological CNS conditions (breaking down to glutamate and aspartate). Choline, on the other hand, is increased with plasma membrane turnover and hence shows increased levels in tumours.

7
Ward Management of Neurosurgical Patients

Jignesh Tailor and Reuben D. Johnson

CONTENTS

INTRODUCTION

Individual Consultants and different neurosurgical units will undoubtedly have their own preferences as to how to manage patients on the ward. However, it is unlikely that the management will differ drastically from that described below. This chapter is designed to give you an overview and an insight into what you are trying to achieve whilst managing patients on the ward. It cannot be overemphasized how important your input is on the ward. The whole unit is built around the nursing staff and the surgical trainees. The calibre of the current batch of surgical trainees is evidenced by how well the unit functions. You should take pride in owning the unit and consider the Registrars and Consultants as mere infrequent visitors – it should never be possible for them to know more about your patients than you do. Good perioperative care really does equate with good outcome.

ADMISSIONS

Most neurosurgical units are busy with a large number of elective and emergency admissions every day. It is essential to be aware of patients who are going to be admitted under your care, so that you can organise your time and prioritise appropriately. There is much that can be done to pre-empt problems and facilitate care before patients arrive on the ward.

EMERGENCY TRANSFERS

Most units will have a list of patients due to come in from other hospitals. Make sure that, at the beginning of each day, you find out from the on-call Registrar which patients are due to come in and what the plan of action for each is. For some patients the plan may be to see and assess, whereas for others it may be that going to theatre is a near certainty unless the patient's condition is radically different from that described by the referring team.

It is recommended that you contact a member of the team looking after each patient in the referring hospital and check up on the patient's situation. A patient might have been on the list for some days and things could have changed considerably. It is useful to ascertain an update on the patient's clinical state and find out what treatment has been initiated. Has the patient with the subarachnoid haemorrhage (SAH) been started on adequate IV fluids? Has the patient with the brain tumour been started on steroids? Has aspirin been stopped on the patient with the posterior fossa tumour due for theatre tomorrow? Has the international normalized ratio (INR) been checked on the patient with the subdural haematoma? Has the sodium been checked recently on the SAH patient?

For a patient being transferred as an emergency, it might be possible to arrange for cross-matched blood to be sent with the patient. For all patients, it is imperative that hard copies of their scans are sent with them. It is usually not possible to print films from an image link, and hard copies of films will be needed in theatre. This is extremely important as it will prevent delays in going to theatre – in neurosurgery, time is life.

The following is a good check-list for a sure and safe transfer:

> S   *Scans*: have hard copies been sent with the patient?
> U   *Update*: has the patient's condition changed?
> R   *Rx*: what treatment has the patient received so far?
> E   *Electrolytes*: are all blood results available?
> &
> S   *Steroids*: have steroids have been given (dose and duration)?
> A   *Aspirin*: if necessary, has aspirin been stopped?
> F   *Fluids*: has appropriate fluid regime been commenced?
> E   *Extra investigations*: CXR? Coag screen? PSA/ESR?

ELECTIVE CASES

It is advisable to make yourself aware of the operating list well in advance. For each patient on the list, make sure they have had a full medical clerking and bloods taken. Patients who have not been assessed in pre-admission clinic may need to be admitted early for a full medical work-up. Make sure you have checked their clotting function and platelet count, and that any blood thinning agents have been stopped. The guidelines for stopping anti-coagulants vary according to the indication for their use and the operation to be performed. In general, aspirin should be stopped 10 days before surgery, warfarin should be reversed on admission 1 to 2 days before surgery, and low molecular weight heparin stopped 48 h before surgery. However, it is essential to know why the patient is on anticoagulants and to liaise closely with the medical team that normally manages the patient. This is particularly important in the case of cardiology patients who may have eluting stents. Find out whether the patient needs any blood saved or cross-matched. In general, an ECG should be performed in all patients with a cardiac history (including hypertension) or who are over the age of 60 years. A preoperative chest X-ray (CXR) should be performed in patients with cardiorespiratory disease (with no CXR in the last 6 months), acute respiratory tract signs or symptoms, malignant disease, or patients who have resided in a tuberculosis endemic area. Alert the anaesthetist to any problems. Find out whether your patient requires any specific preoperative imaging. The neuroradiology department will appreciate knowing this well in advance. Make sure the patient's images are available for the Consultant to view the day before the operation, and that these are also made available in the operating room. You should ask your Registrar or Consultant whether a NICU bed may be required postoperatively, and, if so, give the NICU department plenty of notice, as they are usually very short of beds. The following is a useful check-list for working up elective admissions:

1. History and examination.
2. Blood – FBC, U&E, clotting, G+S or X-match.
3. ECG, CXR (if required).
4. CT/MRI images on the computer system.
5. Preoperative and intraoperative imaging prearranged (if required).
6. HDU/ICU bed prearranged (if required).
7. Anaesthetist review.
8. Consent + site of surgery (SOS) marking by Registrar/Consultant.

GENERAL PRECAUTIONS

In neurosurgery, there are a few basic precautions to keep in mind during your daily tasks, such as prescribing fluids and analgesia. In general, intravenous dextrose solution should be avoided as it can alter the plasma osmolality and increase swelling at the site of intracranial pathology. Normal saline should therefore be used as first-line IV fluid, and in neurosurgery you are allowed to prescribe more than one litre of normal saline in 24 h. You should, however, keep a close eye on the patient's sodium levels, particularly if their renal function is impaired. Neurosurgical patients are also at higher risk of developing abnormalities of sodium due to cerebral salt wasting, the syndrome of inappropriate antidiuretic hormone secretion, and diabetes insipidus, so most patients should have a blood test at least two to three times weekly, unless the patient has suffered a SAH, in which case electrolytes should be checked daily. When prescribing analgesia, you should avoid NSAIDs if possible, particularly if the patient is going to theatre, as this may affect their platelet count. If you are monitoring a neurosurgical patient's level of consciousness, you should prescribe opiates cautiously, as they can make patients feel drowsy and thereby mask any decrease in the level of consciousness due to the underlying intracranial pathology. Finally, ensure that bleeding risk is minimized as much as possible during surgery. This means that you should routinely check that clotting function tests and platelet counts are up to date and clearly documented in the notes, and that any potential blood thinners are avoided in all patients going to theatre. You won't go very wrong if you adhere to the simple CODE of neurosurgical practice:

C *Clotting*: avoid blood thinners before surgery, keep clotting function tests up to date.
O *Opiates*: avoid if monitoring GCS.
D *Dextrose*: avoid in neurosurgical patients; prescribe 0.9% saline.
E *Electrolytes*: watch the sodium!

PERIOPERATIVE CARE
CEREBRAL TUMOURS

Patients with cerebral tumours tend to present with a progressive history of headache, focal neurological deficit, or fits. Patients with signs of raised intracranial pressure or focal neurology will usually benefit from a course of steroids. A loading dose, e.g., 10 mg dexamathasone IV, can be given, followed by 4 mg dexamethasone (oral or IV) qds. This can be gradually reduced after surgery in most instances. If a patient deteriorates whilst on steroids, due to further mass effect of the tumour, it is often worth trying another loading dose of 8–10 mg dexamethasone IV. However, in all cases of neurological deterioration, repeat neuro-imaging must be considered on an urgent basis. Particularly postoperatively, patients are at risk of deteriorating due to increased cerebral oedema or haematoma. If you think the patient's Glasgow Coma Scale (GCS) score has dropped even a point you should inform your Registrar after stabilising the patient and discuss arranging a postoperative CT scan.

It is important to be overcautious with steroids, and to check with the Registrar what the exact plan is. Some patients may have their steroids reduced and stopped while others may be left on a maintenance dose of 2 mg dexamethasone bd orally, at least until seen by the oncologist. Patients cannot be left on steroids indefinitely, and, as a general rule, patients are not usually discharged on steroids unless there is an express instruction from a senior to do so. Steroids have serious side-effects including psychosis, and intracranial or intraspinal sepsis. All patients on steroids need to receive some form of protection against gastric ulceration, e.g., ranitidine or lansoprazole.

In patients with tumours without a tissue diagnosis it is essential to ensure that basic investigations have been performed to rule out a primary lesion outside the CNS. This means that a full history needs to be taken. Has the patient coughed up any blood? Has the patient had any change of bowel habit or passed any blood in the stool? Has the patient had difficulty passing urine? A full clinical examination needs to be performed, including a breast examination in women. A chest X-ray to look for an obvious lung primary is a minimum requirement. Basic blood work should include urea and electrolytes (U&E), full blood count (FBC), liver function tests (LFTs), erythrocyte sedimentation rate (ESR) and clotting studies in the form of an INR. Tumour markers may also be useful in certain patients and include alpha-fetoprotein (testicular cancer), carcino-embryonic antigen (CEA) (colorectal, pancreatic, breast cancers), CA-125 (breast cancer), S-100 (melanoma) and prostate-specific antigen (PSA) (prostate cancer).

Check-list for cerebral tumours

Pre-op
1. Full Hx and Ex for primary tumour.
2. Bloods: FBC, U&E, LFTs, CRP, ESR, clotting studies, tumour markers.
3. CXR
4. Steroids: loading dose (10 mg dexamethasone) and maintenance (4 mg dexamethasone qds).
5. CT scans: done and available on the ward.
6. Operative plan: biopsy/debulk

Post-op
1. Review steroid plan: reduce and stop, or continue maintenance dose.
2. Oncology referral, and liaise with neuropathology regarding histological diagnosis.

SUBARACHNOID HAEMORRHAGE

The ward management of SAH is a fine balance and also extremely important. A good operation is not the only surgical factor that determines a good outcome in SAH. A large part is due to your diligence and meticulous care on the ward. In an ideal world, all SAH patients would be best managed in a high-dependency environment. However, resources being what they are, many patients of good World Federation of Neurosurgeons Scale (WFNS) grade (see Chapter 14, Table 14.3) will, of necessity, be admitted to the neurosurgical ward prior to angiography and surgical treatment. It is important to have a clear idea of the risks these patients face and of what you are trying to achieve perioperatively.

Patients face the greatest risk of a devastating re-bleed in the first 24 h and the risk of re-bleed is as high as 20% in the first 2 weeks following the initial event – with 4% re-bleeding on the first day and 1.5% per day for the next 2 weeks. There is an 80% mortality with a re-bleed. Blood often enters the ventricular system at the time of the initial bleed and patients may develop obstructive hydrocephalus due to blockage of CSF flow within the ventricular system (e.g., aqueduct or outlet of 4th ventricle) or communicating hydrocephalus due to blockage of reabsorption through the arachnoid granulations (this usually occurs at a later stage). If there is a large intraparenchymal blood clot, patients may deteriorate due to the mass effect. SAH patients are at high risk of developing vasospasm, which is one of the major causes of neurological deficit and morbidity in this group (see Chapter 14, Table 14.4). The greatest risk of vasospasm after the initial bleed occurs around 1 week, especially days 4–7; the risk is low in the first 3 days and later than 2 weeks. Electrolyte abnormalities are common in SAH patients

– in particular, hyponatraemia due to cerebral salt-wasting. There is a small but not insignificant risk of seizures developing following SAH. In summary, therefore, you need to be aware that patients admitted with SAH are specifically at risk of:

1. Re-bleeding.
2. Hydrocephalus (usually obstructive in acute phase).
3. Vasospasm/delayed ischaemic neurological deficit (DIND).
4. Hyponatraemia.
5. Seizures.

Your perioperative care is aimed at preventing these complications by reducing the risk of their happening. Measures that need to be taken to prevent re-bleeding include preventing excessive rises in blood pressure. This has to be balanced with preventing an excessive drop in blood pressure which might exacerbate vasospasm. In general, most neurosurgical units will aim to maintain a systolic blood pressure in the range of 120 to 150 mmHg in patients with an unsecured aneurysm. However, this may be difficult to achieve and you may need to seek the help of the NICU team. The patient should be nursed in as quiet and calm an environment as possible, and usually on strict bed rest. Be careful not to put patients in a corner of the ward that is quiet because it is not readily visible – when these patients do deteriorate you will need to act quickly. Patients may be better with 30° head up as, at least in theory, this may help in maintaining CSF flow, reduce intracranial pressure (ICP) due to increased venous return, and prevent chest problems in the more elderly patients. Remember that placing patients on bed rest increases their risk of developing deep-vein thromboses (DVTs), so thromboembolic-deterrent stockings (TEDs) should be prescribed.

Medication is important in preventing large increases in blood pressure, and adequate analgesia should be prescribed, e.g., a codeine phosphate infusion which can be titrated to the clinical response and helps to guard against a precipitous drop in blood pressure associated with some forms of intramuscular analgesia regimes. Antiemetics, and laxatives such as lactulose, help prevent the blood pressure changes associated with nausea and constipation, and should be prescribed. Oral nimodipine has been shown in randomized controlled trials to reduce delayed ischaemic deficits associated with vasospasm. The regime that should be used is 60 mg of nimodipine orally every 4 h, and this should be continued for 21 days after the initial bleed. If patients are unable to take oral medication then an IV infusion can be used instead.

SAH patients should be well hydrated with oral or IV fluids as this is thought to reduce the risk of vasospasm. At least 3 litres of fluid per day should be given; if this is done intravenously, saline is preferable. Hydration is one of the three Hs of 'triple-H' therapy for vasospasm (see Chapter 8 for further discussion). Daily electrolytes should be monitored, with a close eye on the sodium to identify hyponatraemia early.

Routine blood work should include coagulation studies in the form of an INR and group and save (cross-match at least 4 units if the patient is going to have an aneurysm clipped).

Check-list for subarachnoid haemorrhage

1. Strict bed rest.
2. Oral nimodipine 60 mg 4-hourly.
3. 3 litres fluids/day.
4. Analgesia – e.g., codeine phosphate infusion.
5. Antiemetics
6. Lactulose 10 ml bd.
7. U&E, FBC, INR, X-match (daily Na$^+$).
8. Hourly neuro-obs minimum.
9. CT scans available on ward.
10. Results of lumbar puncture (if done) written in notes.
11. CT angiogram or cerebral angiography requested.

HEAD INJURIES

You will see many patients with head injuries during your time as a neurosurgical trainee. In general, if a patient needs admission to a neurosurgical unit then the head injury is severe. Some patients will arrive and go directly to theatre for evacuation of a traumatic bleed (extradural or acute subdural haematomas) or exploration of depressed skull fractures. Others may be unconscious due to diffuse axonal injury or cerebral contusions and will be admitted to the NICU for ICP monitoring and care. There will also be a subgroup of patients with contusions or small intracranial haematomas who are considered at high risk of further deterioration and are, therefore, admitted to the neurosurgical unit for ICP monitoring and observation. If the condition of these patients deteriorates they will need rescanning and either theatre or ICU care.

The principles of head injury care are the same for all patients, and whilst all should have been assessed according to the Advanced Trauma Life Support (ATLS) protocol in the referring hospital, it is nevertheless essential that, on a patient's arrival in the neurosurgical unit, you reassess each patient according to the ATLS protocol, as the patient's situation may have changed.

If a patient is intubated and ventilated, check pupillary response. If bilaterally fixed dilated pupils are found, it may not be appropriate to undertake surgery. If the patient arrives unventilated, then your assessment might determine the need for intubation. Remember: GCS less than 8 = intubate!

If you are not happy with the safety of the airway, speak to your Registrar or the anaesthetist and ask about HDU/ICU care.

Ensure that, if the neck is not immobilized, the patient has had adequate C-spine clearance in the referring hospital. Find the C-spine films and determine whether they are adequate or not. If the patient is not sufficiently awake for clinical assessment of the C-spine do not be afraid to put a collar on the C-spine, even if the neck films are normal. The patient's neck can be reassessed when they are more alert, or by further imaging. Ensure that you are happy with your primary survey before moving on to the secondary survey. If a full trauma series has not been undertaken then ensure that this is done.

Check the notes for blood results – bloods may have been taken but perhaps not checked before transfers. Ensure that you have a sample of blood for cross-match.

Document your neurological assessment clearly to include GCS and pupil reactions. If a patient has deteriorated neurologically at any time, reassess everything again and discuss with the Registrar before sending the patient for another scan. Ask for a minimum of hourly neuro-obs from the nursing staff.

Examine the scalp for wounds and see what management and care they have received. All wounds need to be cleaned properly. If there is an underlying depressed skull fracture, proper surgical exploration and debridement will be required in theatre. Check specifically for CSF leak from the nose and ears and document it.

There are several controversial issues in the management of head injuries. Are anticonvulsants indicated to prevent epilepsy? Should prophylactic antibiotics be given in the presence of CSF leak? Are steroids of any benefit in head injury? All these issues are discussed in Chapter 13 which deals with controversies and evidence base in neurosurgery.

It is generally accepted that prophylactic antibiotics should not be given. If a patient is septic, however, then antibiotics are indicated after appropriate samples have been sent for culture. Discuss with your Registrar regarding choice of antibiotic, and never perform a lumbar puncture (LP) without clearing it with a senior first. If there is an open skull fracture then it is arguable that antibiotics should be given to prevent osteomyelitis.

Steroids are sometimes given, although there is scant evidence for the value of doing so. Again, see the section on controversies in neurosurgery (Chapter 13), and read about the ongoing CRASH (Corticosteroid Randomization After Significant Head Injury) trial. The situation is no more clear-cut for anticonvulsants, but many people will give anticonvulsants prophylactically in the form of phenytoin – this is also discussed in Chapter 13.

The following check-list summarises the actions to be taken in patients admitted with head injury.

Check-list for head injury

1. On arrival in unit, reassess according to ATLS guidelines.
2. If the patient's condition has changed, determine whether they need to be in a HDU/ICU.
3. If the patient is stable, ensure secondary survey complete, including all appropriate radiology (C-spine cleared? – up to 30% of severe head injuries have associated spinal injuries), and ensure all blood work has been done.
4. Document neurology and ensure regular neuro-obs performed.
5. Antibiotics not normally given prophylactically but if there is CSF leak or open skull fracture discuss with Registrar or Consultant.
6. Phenytoin may be given prophylactically, but again discuss preferences with Registrar or Consultant.
7. Steroids probably not indicated.
8. Bloods, including group and save, done.

SHUNT PATIENTS

CSF shunt problems are a common cause for admission to the neurosurgical unit. The commonest problems will be under-shunting of CSF (e.g., due to disconnection or blockage) and infection, although some patients will present with low-pressure headaches due to over-shunting. Patients present in a variety of ways, e.g.: headaches; deterioration in level of consciousness; confusion; focal neurological deficit; sepsis; or fits. Assessment of patients with a shunt problem requires detailed inquiry regarding the history of the shunt itself. What was the indication for the shunt? When and where was it put in? Has it ever needed to be revised, and, if so, which end was revised? Does this episode feel like any previous episodes of shunt problems? Patients usually know if they have a shunt problem; when the patient is a child, always believe the parents – they are almost always right. Enquire about symptoms of raised intracranial pressure (headache, nausea and vomiting, fatigue, ataxia), sources of sepsis (urinary tract infections, respiratory tract infections), and any seizures.

When examining the patient be sure to inspect and palpate the shunt along its entire length, looking particularly for obvious gaps in the shunt and for areas of inflammation. Examine for signs of raised intracranial pressure (papilloedema, VIth nerve palsy, upward gaze palsy, bulging fonatenelles in infants). Pumping and tapping of shunts is best left to the Registrar until you have been taught how to do these. A CT scan needs to be performed and, if possible, old scans should be obtained for comparison. A shunt series of plain films, should be requested, as this provides information about the location of the distal catheter and may identify any obvious disconnections.

Blood work should include white cell count (WCC) and inflammatory markers to look for evidence of an infective process.

Check-list for shunts

1. Full Hx & Ex.
2. CT scan + old films if available.
3. Shunt series.
4. WCC, ESR, CRP.
5. Shunt tap (never do this without discussing with Registrar/Consultant).

PITUITARY PATIENTS

To understand the perioperative care of patients with pituitary tumours it is helpful to consider briefly the effects these tumours may have. The mass effect of pituitary tumours can cause compression of: the optic chiasm, causing visual field defects; the pituitary gland, causing hypopituitarism; and the cavernous sinus, causing compression of cranial nerves III, IV, V_1, V_2, and VI. Pituitary tumours may be functional, secreting a variety of hormones, e.g., prolactin, adrenocorticotrophic hormone (ACTH), growth hormone (GH). It is essential, therefore, to examine and document visual fields and cranial nerves thoroughly. Formal visual field testing by an ophthalmologist is often organized preoperatively and should always be booked postoperatively. Blood work must include endocrine evaluation. Most Consultants will insist that the results of these endocrine investigations are documented in the notes. It is useful to discuss the appropriate blood tests with an endocrinologist early on in your job. Most Consultants will work in liaison with a particular endocrinologist, and getting to know them will greatly facilitate the care of your patients. In general, all pituitary patients will need preoperative assessments of prolactin and growth hormone levels, IgF1, testosterone, follicle-stimulating hormone (FSH), luteinising hormone (LH), and other profiles, to assess their adrenal, gonadal, and thyroid axes. Inducing the pituitary to produce cortisol with an ACTH stimulation test (short synacthen test) will indicate any occult deficiencies in the pituitary secretion of cortisol which might therefore be inadequate during a stress response. These patients need a low maintenance dose of cortisol. There is obviously also a high risk of disrupting pituitary function at surgery, and all patients will need steroid cover postoperatively. An example regime is 100 mg hydrocortisone IV at induction of anaesthesia, followed by 50 mg IV 8–12-hourly postoperatively, reduced gradually to 20 mg mane and 10 mg nocte, both orally, before discharge. Remember to give gastric cover with ranitidine or lansoprazole. Watch carefully for the development of diabetes insipidus (DI) by monitoring urine output and daily sodium levels (see below for management of DI). All pituitary patients need a follow-up endocrinology appointment, and this should be booked and documented in the notes. Prophylactic antibiotics (amoxicillin and flucloxacillin) are commonly given in pituitary surgery as there will be contact of CSF with the nasal cavity. If a CSF leak is detected postoperatively, observe the patient carefully for the development of meningitis and discuss with the Registrar/Consultant about the need for CSF diversion, e.g., lumbar drain.

Check-list for pituitary patients

Pre-op
1. Formal visual field assessment and documentation of cranial nerve examination.
2. Pre-op endocrine assessment discussed with endocrinologist and results documented in notes.
3. Steroid cover from induction and reduced to maintenance post-op.
4. Antibiotic prophylaxis – watch for CSF leak and development of meningitis.

Post-op
1. Monitor urine output and daily Na^+ post-op.
2. Ophthalmology appointment booked.
3. Endocrinology follow-up booked and documented in notes.
4. Monitor for CSF leak.

SPINAL PATIENTS

You will manage a range of spinal patients on the neurosurgical ward, including those with spinal injuries or acute compression syndromes, and patients admitted electively for laminectomies and discectomies. Patients with spinal injuries should be managed in a similar fashion to that described for head-injured patients, with a full reassessment on admission according to ATLS principles. If in doubt about C-spines, ensure that hard collars and sandbags are used. Spinal injury patients are at risk from aspiration and hypotension and so ensure that you are happy with the airway and pay close attention to the blood pressure (minimum IV line with saline infusion). Document the results of a detailed neurological examination, paying particular attention to motor and sensory levels. Document sacral sensation and sphincters (check anal tone and ask whether the patient can feel you pulling gently on their catheter). Steroids may have a role to play in spinal trauma (see Chapter 13 on controversies and evidence in neurosurgery) and methylprednisolone should be given within 8 h of injury – 30 mg/kg over 15 min with a 45 min pause, then 5.4 mg/kg/h for at least the first 24 h (48 h if started >3 h after injury). If a patient needs a fracture stabilized surgically, be sure to check with the operating surgeon regarding instructions for mobilization, e.g., to see whether any check films are required first.

Patients with spinal stenosis or disc prolapse may be admitted electively for surgery, or as an emergency if there is rapidly progressive motor weakness, a cauda equina syndrome or intractable pain. Again, it is important to document neurology, including the presence or absence of saddle anaesthesia and sphincter disturbances. Steroids, in the form of dexamethasone, are advocated in cases of spinal cord compression by some, but not all, neurosurgeons. In the postoperative period it is imperative to document any change in neurology and to check wounds regularly for CSF leak. In patients who undergo anterior approaches through the neck to cervical discs, keep an eye out for haematoma formation as there is a risk of airway compromise with haematomas in the neck. Spinal tumours should be managed in an analogous way to cerebral tumours and these patients will benefit from steroids (dexamethasone).

COMPLICATIONS

If at all possible, it is recommended that you try to attend a course on the management of critically ill surgical patients, as this provides you with a systematic approach to all surgical patients with complications on the ward. The principles are the same for neurosurgery but it is helpful if you are aware of, and understand, some of the complications which are specific to, or common in, neurosurgical patients.

'MRS JONES HAS DIPPED'

This is perhaps the commonest reason you will be called to the ward – because a patient has 'dipped'. Be sure to ascertain what is meant by 'dipped'. It usually refers to a drop in the GCS, or to a deterioration in focal neurology. Go and assess the patient and remember to use an ABCDE approach as neurosurgical patients need system support and can deteriorate from cardiorespiratory problems, such as myocardial infarctions (MIs), pulmonary embolisms (PEs) and chest infections, as much as any other surgical patient. While you are giving oxygen and putting in your lines, find out about the patient's diagnosis and treatment and try to have a list of reasons why a neurosurgical patient might 'dip' neurologically. The following is a useful check-list:

Post-op craniotomy
1. Haematoma – EDH, ASDH, intraparenchymal.
2. Cerebral oedema.
3. Fits.
4. Na^+ abnormalities.
5. Infection – meningitis/abscess.
6. Hydrocephalus

Cerebral tumour patients
1. Further mass effect and oedema.
2. Fits.
3. Bleed associated with tumour.

SAH patients
1. Re-bleed.
2. Hydrocephalus.
3. Vasospasm.
4. Na^+ abnormalities.

Patients with shunts or EVDs
1. Shunt/EVD failure
2. Meningitis
3. Fits

Head injuries
1. Blossoming of contusions.
2. Further bleeding – EDH, ASDH.
3. Fits.
4. Meningitis.
5. Na^+ abnormalities.

Remember to consider rapidly reversible causes, such as low blood glucose and fits. Patients who have fitted may be postictal. Do not be afraid to use lorazepam to control patients who are actively fitting, but beware of using sedatives in patients who are postictal. If in doubt, there is little harm in loading patients with phenytoin (15–18 mg/kg loading dose over at least 30 min to prevent cardiac dysrythmias; maintenance is 5–8 mg/kg/day in single night-time dose or divided doses over the day). Once you are happy that a patient is stable from a cardiorespiratory perspective (this may mean asking the anaesthetist to intubate) then the patient will need some form of repeat imaging, probably in the form of a CT scan. Always inform the Registrar on-call about patients who 'dip' as they may require theatre urgently. Figure 7.1 summarizes the sequence of actions in a patient whose level of consciousness drops on the ward.

CSF LEAKS

CSF leaks may occur after trauma or surgery. CSF leaks from surgical wounds may stop with an extra stitch or two. Patients with CSF leaks following spinal surgery can be placed on bed rest for a few days to reduce the effect of gravity and allow the wound to heal. It is essential to check operative notes and postoperative instructions as there may be a documented breach of the dura at the time of surgery. Antibiotics are not usually given prophylactically for CSF leaks. In patients who develop subcutaneous CSF collections following craniotomy, a lumbar drain is sometimes inserted.

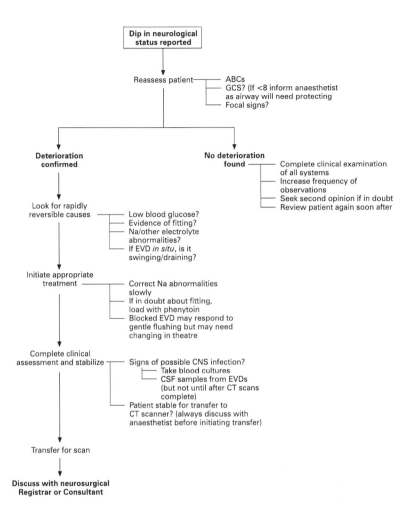

Figure 7.1. Example of the sequence of actions in a patient who 'dips' on the ward, i.e., a deterioration in neurological status is reported. Although there is no single correct sequence of events, this chart highlights various essential points, including the need to consider and, if necessary, treat reversible causes of neurological deterioration before sending a patient to the CT scanner.

Beware being asked to undertake repeated aspirations of CSF collections. There is a significant risk of introducing infection, and if there is no bone flap under the scalp you need to be careful not to damage the brain. There is no right or wrong answer in managing CSF collections, and Consultants will have their own methods based on their own experiences. If a patient with a CSF leak develops signs of sepsis, discuss lumbar puncture and antibiotic treatment with your Registrar or Consultant.

DEEP-VEIN THROMBOSIS

Remember that patients on bed rest are at risk of DVTs and require TEDs and possible anticoagulant prophylaxis. In the neurosurgical population, 30% of patients develop DVTs, although the majority will be asymptomatic.

Check with the Registrar or Consultant before starting anticoagulants, as you need to balance the risk of intradural haematoma with risk of DVT. Most Consultants will be comfortable with anticoagulants more than 48 h after surgery but some may prefer them to be prescribed even sooner. There is literature demonstrating that using low-dose heparin preoperatively and directly postoperatively in craniotomy leads to no increased risk of haemorrhage.

SODIUM ABNORMALITIES

There are several conditions which are frequently seen in neurosurgical patients and which cause abnormalities in serum sodium. You need to be able to recognize them and be familiar with their treatment. Raised serum sodium is seen in diabetes insipidus (DI), and reduced sodium is seen in cerebral salt wasting (CSW) and the syndrome of inappropriate antidiuretic hormone secretion (SIADH). It is particularly important to understand the differences between CSW and SIADH because, although both produce hyponatraemia, they have different effects on extracellular fluid volumes and are treated differently. Remember that all abnormalities of sodium, particularly low sodium, need to be corrected slowly and cautiously due to the risk of central pontine myelinosis. There is an increasing trend for endocrine teams and NICU teams to be involved in the treatment of sodium abnormalities in ward patients.

Diabetes insipidus

Reduced ADH secretion is known as neurogenic DI, whereas renal resistance to ADH is known as nephrogenic DI. Neurogenic DI is the type you are most likely to encounter in neurosurgical patients and may be the result of trauma, tumours, infection, or surgery. Patients at particular risk are those with severe head injury involving damage to the pituitary, after pituitary surgery, or with lesions pressing on the pituitary (e.g., craniopharyngiomas or anterior communicating artery aneurysms). It is important to appreciate that DI may be transient, especially after pituitary surgery. Because of the reduction in ADH there is production of a large volume of dilute urine (>200 ml/h, urine osmolality <200 mosm/l). As a consequence the serum sodium rises (>145 mmol/l with plasma osmolarity >295 mosm/l). In conscious patients this will result in a thirsty patient who classically craves iced water. The volume of fluids taken in may be enough to match losses and keep serum sodium within the normal range. This is where most cases of DI are missed. It is assumed that the high urine output is due to poly-dipsia. The key issue, therefore, is whether or not the kidneys are concentrating urine. A quick bedside test is to dip the urine to test specific gravity. Urine in DI will have a specific gravity <1.005; if it is >1.010, then the patient almost certainly does not have DI. In patients with suspected DI always check specific gravity, serum and urine sodiums and osmolalities. If DI is mild, patients may be able to keep up with fluid losses by taking fluid orally. If DI is more severe, or if the patient is not able to drink because of reduced conscious level, then IV fluids will need to be administered. In this situation dextrose is preferable to saline as the serum sodium is likely to be high. In transient DI, chasing fluid losses until the episode resolves is the best management. However, when it is proving difficult to keep up with losses the ADH analogue 1-d-amino-8-D-arginine vasopressin (DDAVP) may need to be given. This should be used cautiously and only with senior supervision. There is a danger that, if DDAVP is given inappropriately in too high doses, urine output can dry up, with resultant renal shut-down and no urine production, leading to brain swelling and a serious situation. Although the subcutaneous dose is 1–4 μg, we usually start at a lower dose of 0.5 μg or even less.

Cerebral salt wasting

CSW can be defined as renal loss of sodium secondary to intracranial disease. The physiological basis for renal sodium loss is unknown, but it is likely that there is an as yet unidentified natriuretic factor involved. CSW results in hyponatraemia and is also associated with loss of water. This is in contrast to SIADH (see below), in which there is hyponatraemia-associated retention of water due to excess ADH. CSW is seen particularly in patients with SAH. It is essential not to mistake CSW for SIADH in this setting, as fluid restriction (treatment for SIADH) in patients with SAH can precipitate or worsen vasospasm.

To differentiate CSW from SIADH look at the patient's hydration (dry in CSW), central venous pressure (low in CSW), and serum osmolality (normal or high in CSW, low in SIADH). CSW is treated by replacing fluid losses with salt-rich fluids: 0.9% or hypertonic saline. A very effective alternative or adjunctive is fludrocortisone, a mineralocorticoid which may need to be given to stimulate renal reabsorption of sodium; this should, however, be a senior decision, as complications of pulmonary oedema, hypokalaemia and hypertension may occur.

Syndrome of inappropriate antidiuretic hormone secretion

SIADH can occur with a variety of neurosurgical pathology: tumours; head injury; post-craniotomy; meningitis. Inappropriate secretion of ADH results in hyponatraemia due to water retention. Serum sodium and serum osmolalities are therefore low, but there is no detectable abnormality in renal function. Fluid restriction to <1 litre per day is the first-line treatment. The use of hypertonic saline with diuretics should be reserved for refractory cases and undertaken only with senior advice. Remember the warning given above about confusing SIADH and CSW in patients with SAH.

FITS

Fits are a common complication in neurosurgical patients, and patients in status epilepticus need to be stopped from fitting. It is imperative to consider what the cause of the seizure may be, as a patient may have developed a postoperative haematoma that may need surgical evacuation. In status epilepticus, attention must be given to the airway, and oxygen administered. Lorazepam 4 mg IV over 2 min can be given for adults actively fitting. If there is difficulty in obtaining IV access then PR benzodiazepines may be administered. Patients should be loaded with phenytoin 15–18 mg/kg IV over at least 30 min (approx 1 g in a 70 kg adult), even if the lorazepam/diazepam stops the fitting. If fitting still does not stop after phenytoin, call for senior assistance and consider phenobarbitone. Patients who require phenobarbitone to stop fitting generally need a short period on the HDU/ICU where they can be intubated and anaesthetized if necessary. If patients are anaesthetized to control their fits, it is important to obtain a continuous EEG tracing to determine whether or not seizure activity has been controlled – propofol might keep a patient quiet but it may not necessarily stop epileptic activity. Once seizure activity has been controlled, ensure that you initiate the relevant investigations. Check electrolytes and, if the patient was already on phenytoin, check the level. Consider rescanning the patient, as the intracranial picture may have changed, e.g., the development of an extradural haematoma (EDH) after a craniotomy. The basics of managing a fitting patient are summarized in Figure 7.2.

With an isolated fit, consider loading the patient with phenytoin or discuss with a senior regarding alternatives. Again, initiate appropriate investigations and consider rescanning the patient. You may be told about an isolated event consistent with a partial or generalized seizure. Take a good history from the patient or witness, if possible, investigate for any precipitating cause, and consider rescanning the patient if the story is convincing. Starting antiepileptics may have profound social implications for the patient, so you should discuss this with your Registrar or Consultant.

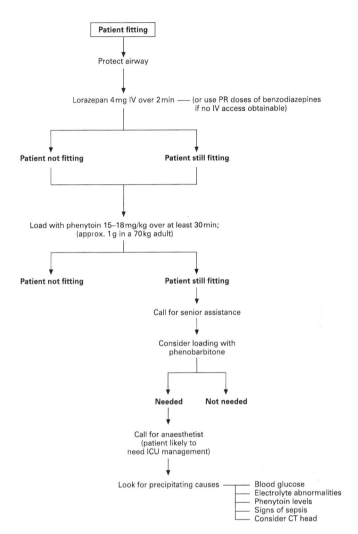

Figure 7.2. Example of management of the fitting patient – doses and protocols may vary locally (NB: doses will be different for paediatric patients – see Chapter 9).

8
Neuro-Intensive Care

Adel Helmy

CONTENTS

INTRODUCTION

The neuro-intensive care unit (NICU) is a vital part of any neurosurgical unit and it is important that all members of the neurosurgical team have an insight into what goes on there – even junior trainees! It may seem a daunting place at first sight, but a methodical approach and a few key principles go a long way to dispelling any of the mystery. The exact role that the basic trainee takes varies from unit to unit; nevertheless every opportunity should be taken to familiarise yourself with the ICU environment. Whilst this chapter cannot turn you into a neuro-intensivist, hopefully it will go some way to allowing you to assess patients, understand the key principles and communicate effectively with your senior colleagues or other specialty teams.

APPROACH TO THE NICU PATIENT

There are many approaches to the ICU patient. Intensivists are fond of amusing acronyms and recommend that you give every ICU patient a 'FAST HUG' every day:

F	**F**eeding
A	**A**nalgesia
S	**S**edation
T	**T**hromboprophylaxis
H	**H**ead up
U	Stress **U**lcer prophylaxis
G	**G**lucose control

This approach is useful, and you can use it if you ever work in ICU. For the assessment of the neurosurgical patient the following ABCDE (Airway, Breathing, Circulation, Disability/neurological assessment, Everything else) approach may be more direct.

AIRWAY

Is the patient's airway protected? Patients with a Glasgow Coma Scale (GCS) score of <9 usually require intubation and ventilation in order to protect their airway. If the patient's clinical state is improving, perhaps this is the time to consider extubating the patient. In the longer term, a patient who cannot maintain their airway may require a tracheostomy. Your anaesthetic colleagues are usually best placed to make these decisions, but it is important for the neurosurgical team to take an active part in this process. Are you expecting the patient to get better or worse? What is the surgical plan for this patient? For example, extubation may be delayed if the patient is expected to go to theatre the following day.

BREATHING

In the awake, spontaneously ventilating patient this assessment is the same as on the ward. In the intubated patient it is important to look at the blood gases and the fractional inspired oxygen concentration (FiO_2). Is the patient's oxygenation improving (FiO_2 coming down) or deteriorating? For example, patients subjected to trauma may have unrecognized chest injuries and patients who have been intubated for some time may develop a chest infection. These factors may prevent a patient from being extubated: usually an FiO_2 of 40% or less is required before extubation is considered. Look carefully at the partial pressure of carbon dioxide (PCO_2). As we shall see, PCO_2 has an important effect on intracranial pressure (ICP).

CIRCULATION

The mean arterial blood pressure (MAP) is an important parameter to check. This pressure is required to perfuse the brain with blood and it may need to be manipulated with fluids and inotropes in patients with raised ICP or vasospasm. The pulse rate can be affected by many factors, such as pyrexia, pain and drugs; however, in the context of trauma a tachycardia is always indicative of blood loss until proven otherwise. Patients with high spinal injuries may have low blood pressure without the normal tachycardic response. This is sometimes called 'neurogenic shock' and it occurs when the sympathethic outflow from the spinal cord (which comes out at thoracic and lumbar levels) is interrupted by spinal cord injury above this level.

DISABILITY/NEUROLOGICAL ASSESSMENT

In the pharmacologically paralysed patient the reaction of the pupils may be the only assessment you can make. This is because both classes of neuromuscular blockers (depolarising and non-depolarising) act at the nicotinic acetylcholine receptor, whilst pupillary constriction is controlled by the parasympathetic nervous system *via* the muscarinic acetylcholine receptor. You should always note both the pupil's size (in mm) and reactivity to light. In patients that are not sedated and paralysed, an assessment of the GCS should be made. It is the most important measure of how patients are progressing. A formal neurological examination can be made if the patient is awake and cooperative; however, a simple assessment of arm or leg movement can be made even in the most uncooperative patient.

EVERYTHING ELSE

This is where FAST HUG comes into its own, to remind you of all the other aspects of managing critically ill patients. Specifically, in the neurosurgical patient, make sure you check their blood glucose, serum sodium, temperature and inflammatory markers. This is not, of course, to say that all the other blood tests are not also important.

SPECIAL TOPICS IN NICU

NICU is a very different environment from the ward, and there are some things you may never have come across before. This section provides an outline of some of the most important.

COMMUNICATION IN NICU

Critically ill patients, such as trauma patients, have pathologies that affect multiple organ systems. This means that many medical teams are involved in their care. At the very least, you will be involved with patients who are jointly under the care of an ICU team (usually anaesthetists) and a neurosurgical team. Communication is absolutely paramount to successfully looking after these complex patients. It avoids conflict and duplication of effort, and it makes the working environment much more pleasant! In ICU, the senior nurses have a wealth of experience and are much better at working things like ventilators and monitors than anyone else. Always hand over any instructions to the nurse looking after the patient, document the plan legibly and include a date, time and signature.

SEDATION AND PARALYSIS

Sedation has many important generic effects, such as reducing pain, anxiety and agitation, and allowing the patient to tolerate a tracheal tube. Together with neuromuscular blockade, sedation helps to increase tolerance to mechanical ventilation and can stop the patient coughing or gagging. More specifically, a wide range of sedative agents reduce neuronal activity. This has the knock-on effect of reducing cerebral metabolism, cerebral blood flow (a phenomenon called flow-metabolism coupling) and intracranial pressure. For these reasons, sedation is widely employed in NICU. The major limitation of sedation to the neurosurgeon is the inability to assess clinically a patient's neurology in order to establish a prognosis or to chart deterioration. For this reason, in sedated patients monitoring techniques such as ICP monitoring are used as an early warning of intracranial insults.

VENTILATION

A detailed discussion of ventilation and mechanical ventilators is outside the scope of this text, but the following principles are important to bear in mind.

Oxygenation

The brain is exquisitely sensitive to hypoxia, and a key requirement in every critically ill patient is to maintain oxygen delivery to the brain. In some patients with associated lung pathology, mechanical ventilation is required to improve oxygenation. In most circumstances, neurosurgical patients require intubation and mechanical ventilation because of their reduced level of consciousness, which means they tend to hypoventilate and fail to protect their airway. In simple terms, there are three methods for improving oxygenation.

1. *Increase the FiO$_2$*: this increases the diffusion gradient across the alveolus.
2. *Increase positive end expiratory pressure*: this keeps alveoli from collapsing at the end of expiration and increases the alveolar surface area available for gaseous exchange.
3. *Increase the inspiratory time: expiratory time ratio:* this works by increasing the time available for gaseous exchange.

Carbon dioxide

There are many factors that control the calibre of the cerebral blood vessels. One of the most important is the PCO$_2$. In normal circumstances, as a part of the brain increases its activity and metabolism it consumes more oxygen and generates more carbon dioxide. In response to the increase in PCO$_2$ the cerebral arterioles relax, dilate and increase the cerebral blood flow. This compensatory mechanism allows an increased delivery of oxygen and metabolic fuels as well as removing more carbon dioxide. This relationship between PCO$_2$ and cerebral-vessel calibre is very important in patients with high ICP. When the PCO$_2$ goes up and the blood vessels dilate this causes an increase in the cerebral blood volume and in ICP. For this reason PCO$_2$ must be kept within tight limits that allow the blood vessels to deliver sufficient oxygen and fuel to the brain without causing too big a rise in ICP. The PCO$_2$ is proportional to the 'minute volume'. This is defined as the amount of gas that moves in and out of the lung in one minute (tidal volume × respiratory rate). The easiest way to control PCO$_2$ on a ventilator is therefore to use a volume control mode. This allows the ventilator to set the tidal volume (the amount of gas pushed into the lung with each breath) and the respiratory rate (the number of breaths per minute). The disadvantage of a volume control mode of ventilation is that the pressure in the lungs is not controlled and in some circumstances can be very high and cause damage.

Tracheostomy

A tracheostomy is a tube that is inserted directly through the anterior part of the neck into the trachea. They come in many types (e.g., cuffed, fenestrated, dual lumen). In NICU they are most commonly used in patients unable to protect their airways for a long period of time, and to aid weaning from mechanical ventilation. It is important to know what they look like and how to replace one in an emergency. It is not uncommon for patients to pull out a tracheostomy, and putting one in quickly can be a life-saving manoeuvre. Patients with a tracheostomy should have suction tubing and forceps available at the bedside for this reason.

INTRACRANIAL PRESSURE MANAGEMENT

A key part of the management of neurological injuries is the prevention of secondary injuries. Different monitoring techniques are used to identify these potential secondary injuries in an effort to prevent them. There are many specialized forms of monitoring that are available on NICU, such as intracranial pressure, jugular venous oximetry, brain tissue oxygen, EEG, microdialysis, transcranial doppler and near infra-red spectroscopy, to name the commonest. Understanding the technicalities of using these monitors, what they measure and how to correct the monitored values when things go wrong, are among the most interesting aspects of managing patients on NICU.

The only monitoring that will be discussed further here is intracranial pressure, as it is the commonest and most important. ICP can be monitored with a dedicated pressure transducer inserted into the skull cavity or *via* an external ventricular drain. The shape and amplitude of the waveform can provide useful information, but it is the mean ICP that is most often used as a goal-directed measure.

ICP monitoring is most commonly used in patients with severe traumatic brain injuries. It serves two important roles. Firstly, it is a monitor for potential deterioration in patients who cannot be assessed clinically because they are sedated and paralysed. Secondly, it acts as a goal-directed target, together with cerebral perfusion pressure (CPP). There is discussion in the literature as to the ideal target for ICP and CPP, but the current consensus is that ICP should be kept below 20 mmHg and CPP should be kept above 60 mmHg. It is absolutely essential to know that these values are for adults, and that the values for babies, infants and young children are completely different (normal intracranial pressure is much lower in a baby than in an adult). It is imperative, therefore, to liaise with your senior colleagues in neurosurgery and in NICU regarding the appropriate values of these parameters for younger patients.

Interpreting ICP properly requires some practical knowledge of the relationship between ICP, CPP and MAP:

$$CPP = MAP - ICP$$

In practice, this means that blood pressure (MAP) is manipulated using fluid therapy and/or inotropes to maintain the CPP, and a number of measures, discussed below, are used to control the ICP. Some neurosurgeons advocate ICP monitoring in other clinical circumstances, but the evidence for this is less clear-cut than for traumatic brain injuries. The following sections discuss the different strategies for controlling ICP. For many of these strategies there are limitations and complications that have to be borne in mind. Balancing the benefit of controlling ICP and the risks of complications from these techniques is difficult in individual patients. Many units use an ICP protocol to help to standardise treatment.

General measures

It is important not to forget simple measures for controlling ICP. The head of the bed should be raised by 30° to aid venous drainage, and tracheal tapes and a cervical collar should be well fitting to avoid compression of the neck veins. Body temperature should be kept below 37°C with antipyretic agents such as paracetamol, or by active cooling if necessary. In addition, any seizures should be treated with an antiepileptic agent.

Surgical management of ICP

It may seem obvious, but in patients with high ICP any intracranial mass lesions should be considered for evacuation. Mass lesions include haematomas (extradural, subdural or intraparenchymal) and contusions. In addition, there are two other surgical methods for reducing ICP: extra-ventricular drainage of CSF and decompressive craniectomy.

An extraventricular drain (EVD) can be useful, because some patients will develop hydrocephalus following a head injury; however, even if there is no hydrocephalus present, draining any residual intracranial CSF will reduce ICP. Some centres use continuous drainage of CSF and some use intermittent drainage, but the principle is the same. The disadvantage of using this technique is that the patient is subjected to a surgical procedure and the risk of EVD infection, particularly if the drain is kept in for more than 5 days.

Decompressive craniectomy is an alternative approach and involves removal of a large section of the skull vault to increase the volume of the intracranial space. This can be done laterally, bifrontally or over the posterior fossa, and is often combined with an operation to remove any intracranial mass lesion. It is a very effective method for controlling ICP but has the risks of a craniotomy, and sometimes there are problems with kinking of cerebral veins at the edge of the craniectomy where the brain bulges out. In addition, if patients survive, many will request a cranioplasty in order to correct the defect, with the risks of a further operation.

Sedation and paralysis

As already discussed, sedation reduces neuronal activity, cerebral blood flow and cerebral blood volume. Paralysis stops the patient from 'fighting' the ventilator and this reduces intrathoracic pressure. Intrathoracic pressure is transmitted to the intracranial cavity *via* the venous system, and can increase ICP. These two interventions are very effective; however, prolonged sedation and paralysis make the patient prone to chest complications, particularly infection.

Hyperosmolar agents

Mannitol and hypertonic saline (e.g., 5%) are used when it is necessary to control ICP rapidly, as when a patient develops a fixed, dilated pupil.

Traditionally, the explanation for their action is that they cannot get across the blood-brain barrier and therefore exert an osmotic gradient across the blood-brain barrier which draws fluid from the brain. Although this is undoubtedly true, they act too quickly on ICP for this to be the only mechanism involved. Other theories regarding the mechanism of action include improvement of the rheology (resistance characteristics) of blood by causing a transient increase in blood volume, or dehydration of red blood cells and a reduction in their volume, thus allowing them to pass through the microcirculation better; in addition, mannitol may have a free radical effect.

The limitation of hyperosmolar agents is that they cause a progressive increase in serum sodium concentration and osmolarity. Mannitol, which is a diuretic, can also cause severe hypokalaemia. The major practical difference between hypertonic saline and mannitol is that hypertonic saline is a volume expander and mannitol is a diuretic. In patients with polytrauma and hypotension, hypertonic saline is the more useful when available.

Hyperventilation

As discussed in the section on ventilation, the PCO_2 is a major determinant of cerebral vessel tone and therefore of ICP. There is a trade-off between keeping the PCO_2 down to decrease ICP and keeping it high enough to maintain cerebral blood flow and thus stop the brain from becoming ischaemic. For this reason, hyperventilation is not recommended outside the setting of NICU, where specialist monitoring, such as jugular oximetry or brain tissue oxygen, can be used to make sure that hyperventilation is not making the brain ischaemic. In NICU the PCO_2 is kept in the lower normal range (4.5–5 kPa) unless there is a particularly refractory ICP, when it can be taken as low as 4 kPa, bearing in mind the provisos above.

Therapeutic hypothermia

Hypothermia below a temperature of 37°C can be used to reduce neuronal activity, cerebral blood flow, cerebral blood volume and ICP. Progressive hypothermia inhibits cardiac and renal function and makes patients, particularly if elderly, susceptible to infection. For this reason, active cooling is used with caution and patients are not usually cooled below 33°C.

Barbiturates

The barbiturate class of drugs, e.g., thiopentone or pentothal, are powerful sedatives. They are not usually used as first-line sedative drugs because they can inhibit cardiac function and cause problems with potassium homeostasis. They are, however, sometimes used when other management strategies have failed. The RESCUEicp study (www.rescueicp.com) is a multi-centre randomized study comparing barbiturates with decompressive craniectomy for patients with intractable rises in ICP.

MANAGEMENT OF VASOSPASM

Vasospasm refers to constriction of the cerebral blood vessels which most commonly occurs following aneurysmal subarachnoid haemorrhage (SAH). However, it can occur following any cause of SAH, including trauma. It typically begins 4–7 days following SAH and can present with any number of neurological deficits, from a focal deficit to a reduction in GCS. Although vasospasm was first described as a phenomenon of the large cerebral vessels seen on cerebral angiography, the neurological deficits following SAH do not always coincide with angiographic vasospasm. The pathophysiology of the clinical syndrome which is commonly referred to as vasospasm is, therefore, more accurately referred to as a delayed ischaemic neurological deficit (DIND). This term reflects the fact that the underlying pathophysiology is likely to be more complex than simple spasm of the large cerebral arteries. Nonetheless, vasospasm is the most commonly used term to refer to DIND and so these terms will be used here interchangeably. The pathophysiology of vasospasm relates to the blood load within the subarachnoid space: vasospasm is more common as the blood load increases. The severity of blood load as seen on a CT scan has been graded by Fisher (see Table 14.4 in Chapter 14) and a Fisher grade 3 has the highest risk of vasospasm at ~70%. Vasospasm is a significant cause of morbidity and mortality in patients who survive the first few days following an SAH. All patients admitted with a diagnosis of SAH are kept on oral nimodipine 60 mg 4-hourly for 21 days, to reduce the risk of vasospasm (British Aneurysm Nimodipine Trial) and are kept well filled with intravenous fluids, typically 3 litres of normal saline per day.

Diagnosis and investigation

Despite these treatments, a proportion of patients will develop a DIND. In order to clinch a diagnosis of vasospasm three things are required: (1) a consistent clinical picture of an unexpected clinical deterioration 4–20 days following SAH; (2) exclusion of alternative diagnoses, and (3) ideally, evidence of hypoperfusion of the relevant cortical area. Alternative diagnoses may include hydrocephalus, re-bleed, electrolyte disturbance (especially hypo- and hyper-natraemia), seizures, sepsis and hypoglycaemia. Typical investigations are CT Head scan, a full set of bloods, EEG (if available) and a thorough clinical assessment. There is no single foolproof investigation for diagnosing vasospasm. The best investigation is cerebral angiography, but it is invasive and cannot be repeated too frequently. Trans-Cranial Doppler (TCD) is a method for assessing the velocity of blood flow in a major branch of the Circle of Willis, usually the anterior or middle cerebral arteries. The principle behind its use is that the narrower the vessel calibre, the higher the absolute velocity of blood within the vessel. This velocity does not take into account the flow within the vessel: if the flow increases then the velocity of blood flow will increase without a change in vessel diameter. To correct for this the Lindegaard ratio (LR) is used: this is the ratio of flow velocities within the middle cerebral artery (MCA) and the extracranial internal carotid artery (EICA):

$$LR = \frac{\text{flow velocity within the MCA}}{\text{flow velocity within the EICA}}$$

An LR ratio of >3 is used for the diagnosis of vasospasm. TCD is useful in the unconscious patient, where it can be repeated on a daily- or twice-daily basis. With repeated measurements, the trend of TCD measurements is most informative. Newer imaging techniques, such as perfusion CT scan, are being used increasingly to demonstrate the hypoperfusion associated with vasospasm.

Treatment of vasopasm

The treatment of vasospasm is summarized as 'triple-H'. The three Hs are:

Hypertension: to increase the flow of blood through the narrowed vessel.

Haemodilution: to improve the rheology of blood by reducing blood viscosity.

Hypervolaemia: to increase cardiac output through the Frank-Starling mechanism.

Triple-H therapy can be used only in patients who have their aneurysm secured, as clearly hypertension can increase the risk of aneurysmal re-bleed. In practice, the patient has a central venous catheter and arterial line inserted for monitoring. Fluids are used to increase the central venous pressure to the upper limit of normal (10–12 mmHg) and to reduce the haematocrit to 30–40%. If the patient's neurological deficit does not improve then inotropes (such as noradrenaline) can be used to push up the blood pressure. Typically, the MAP can be pushed up to 100–120 mmHg; however, if this does not work, some authors recommend raising the MAP further. Hypertensive therapy can precipitate cardiac ischaemia and should be used with caution in the elderly or in those with a previous history of ischaemic heart disease.

In a proportion of patients, the neurological deficit persists despite triple-H therapy, and can eventually lead to cerebral infarction and an irreversible deficit. In this circumstance, angiographic intervention with angioplasty or intra-arterial vasodilators (such as nimodipine or papaverine) can be considered; the benefits, however, may be only short-lived.

BRAIN HERNIATION SYNDROMES

The definition of a hernia from general surgery is 'the protrusion of a viscus through the wall which normally contains it, into an abnormal situation'. An analogous situation can happen in the intracranial compartment. In this circumstance, the dural leaves making up the tentorium cerebelli and falx cerebri divide the skull cavity into left and right supratentorial compartments and the posterior fossa. If there is a localized increase in pressure in any of these compartments, brain tissue can be forced out. When any cerebral herniation occurs, three things need to be considered:

1. What is herniating?
2. Where is it herniating?
3. What is compressed? (This will tell you what the clinical consequences will be.)

Compression of a cerebral artery leads to ischaemia or infarction in the relevant vascular territory. In transtentorial herniation, compression of the midbrain leads to a fixed, dilated pupil (third nerve nucleus), hemiparesis (cerebral peduncle) and coma (periacqueductal grey). The lateralising signs are usually ipsilateral to the side of the compression, but occasionally the entire midbrain is pushed over and is compressed at the tentorial incisura on the other side, leading to contralateral clinical signs. The eponym for the tentorial incisura is 'Kernohan's notch' and for this reason the phenomenon of contralateral signs with transtentorial herniation is called Kernohan's phenomenon and is said to occur in 10% of cases. Transtentorial herniation can also be of the cerebellar vermis upwards through the tentorial incisura if there is a posterior fossa mass. Tonsillar herniation is a rapidly fatal event, as the cardiorespiratory homeostatic centres are within the medulla. Cushing's phenomenon is bradycardia and hypertension associated with tonsillar herniation. It is a consequence of medullary ischaemia, causing a surge of sympathetic activity with a reflex bradycardia mediated by the parasympathetic nervous system. It is not a clinically useful sign of raised intracranial pressure as it occurs very late and, by this time, the patient is inevitably in deep coma. A summary of herniation syndromes can be seen in Table 8.1

BRAIN STEM DEATH

Brain stem tests are a sequence of clinical tests to evaluate brain stem function. In the UK, if a patient meets the criteria for brain stem death on this basis they are legally dead. This has particular relevance to neurosurgeons as there are many cerebral pathologies that are irrecoverable but will allow a patient's heart to continue beating whilst they are on a ventilator. There is also an implication for transplant surgeons as a proportion of organ donors will come from these unfortunate patients, so called 'beating heart' donors.

Table 8.1. Common cerebral herniation syndromes.

Herniation	What	Where	Compressed
Subfalcine	Cingulate gyrus	Below the falx cerebri between the two supratentorial compartments	Anterior cerebral artery
Transtentorial	Uncus of the temporal lobes	Through the tentorial incisura	Midbrain posterior cerebral artery
Tonsillar	Cerebellar tonsils	Through the foramen magnum	Medulla oblongata

This is of great value to transplant recipients as the organ's ischaemic time is minimized. The legal situation differs in other countries; for example, in the USA, EEG and angiographic findings are also used.

For a patient to be pronounced brain stem dead two sets of criteria need to be met, as discussed below. The tests themselves must be carried out by two experienced doctors of at least 5 years standing. Usually they are carried out by intensive care and neurosurgical consultants. The tests must be done by each of the doctors, but this can occur at the same time. If there is a period of time between the two tests it is the time of the first set of tests that is taken as the legal time of death, although this cannot be verified until the second set of tests. The patient's friends and relatives need to be counselled carefully regarding brain stem death as it is a difficult time for them and the purpose and legal implications of the tests can seem confusing.

Prerequisites

Before the actual brain stem tests are carried out, a number of prerequisites must be met:

1. The patient must not be under the influence of any sedative or paralysing drugs.
2. The patient must not have any systemic disturbance that could cause coma, and must
   a. be normothermic; and
   b. have normal serum biochemistry.
3. Apnoeic coma
   a. The patient must have a GCS of 3, despite persistent stimulus in the dermatome of the trigeminal nerve (usually over the supra-orbital notch);
   b. The patient must be apnoeic. This test is done by pre-oxgenating the patient and passing a tube carrying high flow

oxygen down the endotracheal tube to maintain oxygenation. The ventilator is then switched off to allow the PCO_2 to rise. The patient's chest is uncovered to ensure that there is no respiratory effort. Before the test is completed a blood gas must be taken to ensure that the PCO_2 has reached at least 8 kPa. This level of hypercarbia should stimulate the respiratory centres.

Brain stem tests

To meet the criteria for brain stem death the patient must also have no brain stem function. The following tests are designed to test the brain stem. You should think of each of the following tests in terms of the afferent and efferent limbs, and the part of the brain stem in which the relevant cranial nuclei reside (see Table 8.2).

Table 8.2. Summary of brain stem tests.

Test	Afferent limb	Efferent limb	Site of brain stem nuclei
Pupillary light reflex	II	III	Midbrain
Corneal reflex	Va	VII	Pons
Doll's eye reflex	VIII	III/VI	Pons/midbrain
Caloric reflex	VIII	III/VI	Pons/midbrain
Gag reflex	XI/X	XI/X	Medulla

1. *Pupillary light response*. The pupils must be fixed, dilated and unresponsive to light.
2. *Corneal reflex*. The patient must not blink when a wisp of cotton is drawn across the cornea.
3. *Doll's eye reflex*. The eyes are held open and the head is turned from side to side. The patient's eyes must not move. This is also called the vesitubulo-ocular reflex.
4. *Caloric testing*. Otoscopy is carried out to ensure that the external auditory meatus is free of any obstruction. Ice-cold water is slowly instilled into the outer ear. This procedure leads to convection currents within the semi-circular canals which normally lead to the eyes deviating towards the ear in which the water is instilled. No response is seen if the patient is brain stem dead.
5. *Gag reflex*. The endotracheal tube is pulled or a suction catheter is placed down the tube to stimulate the pharynx. No cough or gag should be seen.

9
Paediatric Neurosurgery
Saurabh Sinha and Reuben D. Johnson

CONTENTS

Ward-based management
General work up
Further treatment
Paediatric brain tumours
Pilocytic astrocytoma
Pathophysiology
Epidemiology
Treatment
Outcome
Primitive neuroectodermal tumours
Pathophysiology
Epidemiology
Treatment
Outcome
Ependymoma
Pathophysiology
Epidemiology
Treatment
Outcome
Choroid plexus papilloma and carcinoma
Pathophysiology
Epidemiology
Treatment
Outcome
Brainstem gliomas
Clinical features of paediatric brain tumours
Management of paediatric brain tumours
General work up
Specific work up
Treatment options
Follow-up imaging

OVERVIEW OF PAEDIATRIC PATIENTS

Whilst it is beyond the remit of this book to deal with the entire topic of paediatric neurosurgery, there are important aspects that can be highlighted. For many trainees in surgical specialties, there may have been little or no contact with paediatric patients. We have therefore included a brief overview of some important physiological aspects at the beginning of this chapter. We have then given our view of how paediatric patients may best be evaluated. It is essential to remember that, in the care of any critically ill child, the mandatory management involves optimization of airway, breathing and circulation (ABC) prior to any attempts at definitive care. In the later parts of this chapter we will consider several aspects of clinical paediatric neurosurgery with which we feel new trainees should be familiar, including hydro-cephalus, head injuries, and paediatric brain tumours.

HOW DO CHILDREN DIFFER FROM ADULTS AND FROM EACH OTHER?

The management of children is complicated by their differences from adults, and also by their own diversity. Some of the main ways in which these differences occur are discussed below.

Weight

A child's weight increases most rapidly during the first year of life. At birth, the average weight is 3.5 kg and this rapidly rises to 10 kg at 1 year. The rate of increase slows until puberty when there is often another rapid rise. Fluid and drug therapies as well as blood volume in children are guided by weight, and therefore an accurate weight is essential for optimal management. An estimated weight can be obtained using the following formula:

$$\text{Weight (kg)} = 2 \times (\text{age in years} + 4)$$

Fluids

- Circulating blood volume = 80 ml/kg (60 ml/kg in adults)
- Fluid bolus for resuscitation = 20 ml/kg crystalloid
- Transfusion of packed cells = 10 ml/kg
- Transfusion of whole blood = 20 ml/kg
- Maintenance fluids over 24 h = 100 ml/kg (first 10 kg); 20 ml/kg (next 10 kg); 10 ml/kg after that.

Anatomy

The proportion of head to body size is significantly increased in infants in comparison with adults. The infant brain reaches approximately 75% of its adult size by 18 months of age and accounts for just over 10% of total body weight. Children lose a significant proportion of heat from the head and the increased head-to-body ratio (19% of body surface area at birth) can lead to a rapid loss of heat and leave them prone to hypothermia.

Physiology

Children are born with a small cardiorespiratory reserve and an immature immune system. Infections such as meningitis are, therefore, more of a concern in babies than in older children. Maternal antibodies crossing the placenta provide some protection, but this diminishes over the first 6 months. The physiological changes that occur as children grow mean that there are significant changes to heart rate, blood pressure and respiratory rate with age (see Table 9.1). The presence of open fontanelles and their subsequent closure, as well as the increase in CSF production as children grow leads to differences in their intracranial pressure (ICP). The range of ICP in

119

infants is approximately 3–8 mmHg and rises towards 15 mmHg after the fontanelle closes.

With the associated changes in blood pressure (mean arterial pressure in newborn is around 50 mmHg rising to 80 mmHg in mid-teens), cerebral perfusion pressure (CPP) may only be 40–50 mmHg in infants, and nearer to 70 mmHg in teenagers.

Table 9.1. Change in vital signs with age.

Age (years)	Heart rate (beats/min)	Systolic blood pressure (mmHg)	Respiratory rate (breaths/min)
<1	110 – 160	70 – 90	30 – 40
1–2	100 – 150	80 – 95	25 – 35
2–5	95 – 140	80 – 100	25 – 30
5–12	80 – 120	90 – 110	20 – 25
>12	60 – 100	100 – 120	15 – 20

Psychology

Communication can be a difficult problem with infants and young children, The lack of complex language function often prevents description of their symptoms and may require help *via* nonverbal information. Older children will have a better understanding, and anxiety can be eased by appropriate communication. Fear and anxiety often accompany illness and injury in children, and can significantly alter their cardiorespiratory indices, making clinical assessment difficult. Providing them with age-appropriate information can help to allay some of their fears and to establish a rapport.

TAKING A PAEDIATRIC HISTORY

It is always useful to take as much information from the child as possible. Often they will tell you important features that family members may not have noticed, especially if the symptoms are chronic in nature. It also helps to establish a relationship with the child; this often eases any anxiety in both the child and the parents. The key aspects of a paediatric history are as follows:

- *Pregnancy and delivery*: infections and illness during pregnancy and complications during delivery can lead to a variety of neurological insults. Prematurity increases the risk of intraventricular haemorrhage and subsequent hydrocephalus.

- *Development/schooling*: inability to attain developmental milestones, or new difficulties with schoolwork, may be the only indications of an ongoing neurological problem.

- *General behaviour*: young children with raised intracranial pressure may present with altered sleeping patterns, worsening temper and 'head-banging'.

- *Other siblings*: developmental milestones in siblings may allow comparison with the affected child.

- *Developmental milestones*: these are shown in Table 9.2.

GENERAL EXAMINATION

Examination of older cooperative children is essentially similar to that of adults. In younger children, it is not always possible to carry out a full neurological examination, and varying strategies may need to be adopted to obtain a useful assessment. Don't forget the role of the parents: it may be more reassuring to the child to be examined on their parent's lap. As with adult patients, general inspection provides essential information, and the following list of questions should go through your mind during the examination:

(1) Are there dysmorphic features?

- Craniofacial dysmorphism may suggest a diagnosis of craniosynostosis.

(2) Are there significant cutaneous features?

- Don't forget to examine the midline!
- Cutaneous signs can give important clues to the underlying diagnosis, e.g., café-au-lait spots and neurofibromas are seen in neurofibromatosis, facial port wine stains in Sturge-Weber syndrome.
- Midline deformities such as a sacral dimple and cleft palate may also provide important clues to underlying pathology.

(3) Is the child alert/playful/interactive? Are they easy to handle?

- Children with acute neurological disturbance are often irritable and difficult to handle This may be the only feature that a parent notices.

(4) Is the anterior fontanelle soft and pulsatile or tense and bulging? Are the scalp veins distended or flat?

- A tense, bulging fontanelle is suggestive of raised intracranial pressure, especially if it remains as the head is raised.
- The presence of distended scalp veins is a further feature suggestive of raised intracranial pressure.

Table 9.2. Developmental milestones.

Age	Motor skills	Language skills	Social skills	Concerns
6 weeks	Pull to sit. Head lags Fixates and follows to 90°	Vocalises Quiets or startles to sound	Smiles responsively	Failure to fix/follow visually No response to sound Doesn't smile Asymmetric reflexes
3 months	Follows object (180°) Grasp object placed in hand	Turns head to sound Squeals with delight	Laughs	
6 months	Rolls Sits up Reaches for objects	Babbles	Mouthing Feeds self with biscuit	
9 months	Pulls self to stand Simple pincer grip	Understands 'No'	Stranger anxiety	Unable to sit Hand preference Limited 'babble'
12 months	Stands a one Walks with support	One/two words with meaning Understands simple phrases	Waves 'bye-bye' Plays 'peek-a-boo'	
18 months	Gets up/down stairs with support Handedness	More words Points to objects wanted	Feeds self with cup/spoon	Unable to walk/stand unsupported Inability to understand simple commands No spontaneous vocalization No pincer grip
24 months	Runs Kicks a ball Makes a tower of several Cubes	2–3 words into sentence Uses 'you' and 'me'	Puts on shoes Dry by day Plays near other children	
3–5 years	Stands on one foot Skips Hops	Count to 10 Names colours Knows age	Plays with others Dresses/undresses Dry by night	Unable to speak in short sentences Unable to colour match

(5) Is there failure of upward gaze ('sun-setting')?

- This is another feature suggestive of raised intracranial pressure often secondary to hydrocephalus, and is due to pressure on the tectal plate. It can, therefore, also be seen with tumours in this region, e.g., pineal tumours.

KEY ASPECTS OF THE NEUROLOGICAL EXAMINATION

LEVEL OF CONSCIOUSNESS

In critically ill children it is often important to obtain a quick overview of the problematic systems after the primary resuscitation. The AVPU scale allows for a rapid brief assessment of the overall level of consciousness.

- A   **A**lert
- V   Responds to **V**oice
- P   Responds to **P**ain
- U   **U**nresponsive

If a more formal assessment is required, the Glasgow Coma Scale (GCS) can be used in its modified paediatric form. The key differences are shown in Table 9.3.

Table 9.3. Key differences in the paediatric GCS from the adult GCS.

Eyes	Verbal	Motor
Unchanged (as for adult GCS)	5 – smiles, coos, babbles 4 – cries, irritable but consolable 3 – cries to pain, occasionally consolable 2 – moans to pain, inconsolable, agitated 1 – none	6 – spontaneous or purposeful movements

TONE AND REFLEXES

It is often easier to assess power and coordination by observing the child 'playing'. Ask the child to skip/hop/jump/run. Not only does this provide useful knowledge but makes the examination fun for the child, thereby diminishing their anxiety about future visits. Young children are always keen on trying to copy their favourite characters; e.g., girls love to pretend to be Angelina Ballerina and will attempt to carry out complex twirls. Generalized reflexes are usually elicitable after 33 weeks gestation. Although there are some differences in both tone and reflexes in children, the lack of symmetry should alert you to a potential neurological disorder. Hypertonicity in the flexors of the elbow, hip and knees is not abnormal in the first few months. The tone in the ankles may be markedly reduced whilst remaining normal in other joints. Children <2 years have an extensor response (Babinski) in their great toe and this is a normal feature. Some of the primitive reflexes are shown in Table 9.4.

Table 9.4. Primitive reflexes.

Reflex	Description
Grasp reflex	Present until about 6 months
Moro reflex	Also known as the 'startle' response, this reflex is present until about 4 months
Landau reflex	In the prone position, with the abdomen supported, the head should extend and the hips flex (if no lower limb abnormalities)
Rooting reflex	Stimulation around the mouth should lead to turning of the head to the stimulated side

PAEDIATRIC HYDROCEPHALUS
CSF PHYSIOLOGY

Cerebrospinal fluid (CSF) is considered a part of the transcellular fluids. It is contained in the ventricles and the subarachnoid space, and bathes the brain and spinal cord. The CSF is contained within the meninges and acts as a cushion to protect the brain from injury resulting from position or movement. The CSF is formed by modified ependymal cells in the choroid plexus and directly from the walls of the ventricles. It is absorbed by the arachnoid villi and directly into cerebral venules. There is experimental evidence to suggest that CSF may also flow along the cranial nerves and spinal nerve roots, allowing it into the lymphatic channels; this flow may play a role in CSF reabsorption in neonates, in whom there are few arachnoid granulations.

In adults and older children the total volume of CSF is 150 ml. The daily production is approximately 500 ml/day so the CSF turns over about three to four times per day. Experimental evidence suggests that CSF production in infants is approximately 125 ml/day, rising to about 320 ml/day by the age of 2 years.

The CSF has a composition identical to that of the brain extracellular fluid (ECF), but this is different from plasma. The major differences from plasma are:

- PCO_2 is higher (50 mmHg), resulting in a lower CSF pH (7.33).
- Protein content is normally very low (0.2 g/l), resulting in a low buffering capacity.
- Glucose concentration is lower.
- Chloride concentration is higher.
- Cholesterol content is very low

There are no lymphatic channels in the brain, and CSF fulfills the role of returning interstitial fluid and protein to the circulation. The CSF is separated from blood by the blood–brain barrier. Only lipid-soluble substances can easily cross this barrier, and this is important in maintaining the compositional differences.

CONGENITAL HYDROCEPHALUS

Hydrocephalus is the most common reason for admitting children to a neurosurgical unit. Hydrocephalus in children, as in adults, can be communicating or noncommunicating. The commonest causes are:

- Post-haemorrhagic (premature infants, intraventricular haemorrhage).
- Post-infective (usually after meningitis).
- Aqueductal stenosis.
- Dandy-Walker syndrome.
- Chiari malformation (usually associated with spina bifida).
- In association with tumours (e.g., posterior fossa, choroid plexus, third ventricle, pineal).

It is important to have some knowledge of the different causes of congenital hydrocephalus.

Myelomeningocoele

Approximately 80% of patients born with a myelomeningocoele have an associated problem with hydrocephalus. Although the initial concern is with the spinal defect, following closure the majority of these children will require treatment for hydrocephalus. Magnetic resonance images (MRI) of the neural axis should be obtained when the child is well, as these children commonly have an associated Type II Chiari malformation.

Aqueduct stenosis

This condition accounts for approximately 10% of congenital hydrocephalus. It can be secondarily acquired due to gliosis around the periaqueduct following intrauterine infections or haemorrhage. Four variants exist, all of which cause some form of narrowing of the aqueduct: *gliotic variant*, with narrowing caused by proliferation of subependyal astrocytes; *forking variant*, with several channels separated by normal tissue (associated with spina bifida); *septal variant*, with a septum across the aqueduct; and *true narrowing*, in which the aqueduct is histologically normal but has a narrow diameter.

Intraventricular haemorrhage

Approximately 35% of premature infants who have suffered an intraventricular haemorrhage (IVH) will go on to develop hydrocephalus. The increased survival of very premature infants with improvements in neonatal care make this an increasingly important cause of congenital hydrocephalus. Haemorrhage usually occurs in the germinal matrix within the first 3 days of life. The IVH severity scale is presented in Table 9.5. The underlying pathophysiology is not entirely understood. However, the walls of blood vessels in the germinal matrix region lack certain structural elements present in more mature vessels in the premature neonate. Furthermore, the germinal matrix is the site of origin for cortical neuronal and glial cells. The blood vessels in this region are therefore required to provide sufficient blood for these rapidly dividing cells. These fragile vessels are exposed to significant changes in arterial and venous pressures in the premature infant, and this can lead to rupture and haemorrhage.

Table 9.5. Intraventricular haemorrhage (IVH) severity scale.

Grade	Features
I	Germinal matrix haemorrhage without extension into the ventricle
II	IVH involving up to 50% of ventricular area and not dilating the ventricle
III	IVH involving greater than 50% ventricular area and dilating the ventricle
IV	Intraparenchymal component outside the germinal matrix region

X-linked hydrocephalus

This is an inheritable form of aqueductal stenosis found only in male children. It constitutes fewer than 4% of all cases and accounts for 8–15% of primary hydrocephalus in boys. The underlying genetic anomaly is the presence of an abnormal gene located on Xq28, leading to a deficiency of the L1 cell adhesion molecule. It is commonly associated with mental retardation, corpus callosum hypoplasia, adducted thumbs and lower limb spasticity.

Dandy-Walker malformation

Dandy-Walker malformation (DWM) accounts for approximately 2–4% of congenital hydrocephalus. It is characterized by atresia of the foramina of Lushka and Magendie, partial or total agenesis of the cerebellar vermis and cystic dilatation of the fourth ventricle with a subsequent enlargement of the posterior fossa. 70–90% of patients with DWM develop hydrocephalus. The condition is often associated with other developmental anomalies including cranial and spinal dysraphism, dysgenesis of the corpus callosum and cardiac anomalies. Hydrocephalus treatment in DWM involves shunting of the fourth ventricle +/- lateral ventricles. Standard ventricular-peritoneal shunting may lead to upward herniation and should not be used in isolation. A formal cardiac assessment is required prior to surgical intervention. The long-term prognosis is dependent on the absence or presence of other anomalies. When DWM is present in its mildest form, patients may remain undiagnosed until much later in life.

MANAGEMENT OF PAEDIATRIC HYDROCEPHALUS

Presenting features

Older children may present with the usual features of raised intracranial pressure: headache (usually worse in the morning or on lying down); vomiting; and double/blurred vision. More subtle presenting features include a deterioration in schoolwork and behavioural changes. Parinaud's Syndrome (failure of upward gaze, light-near dissociation) and papilloedema may be seen. Younger children may present with an increasing head circumference, developmental delay, poor feeding and/or failure to thrive, irritability and poor handling, or sleep disturbances. A bulging fontanelle, distended scalp veins, occipito-frontal circumference >98th centile, and sunsetting eyes may be seen.

Treatment

* Don't forget: the treatment of *all* critically ill children starts with ABC!

General work up

* *U&Es*: vomiting leads to electrolyte imbalance and dehydration.
* *FBC*: signs of infection.
* *Coagulation screen*: if presenting with haemorrhage.
* *Group and Save.*
* *TORCH screening in newborn*: **TO**xoplasmosis, **R**ubella, **C**ytomegalovirus, **H**erpes simplex are infections that can get passed from mother to foetus and can lead to focal cerebral calcification and hydrocephalus.
* *IV cannulation and fluids*: bolus 10 ml/kg if dehydrated.
* *CT scan*: to assess ventricular size and anatomy, haemorrhage and space-occupying lesions.
* *MRI*: allows better demonstration of ventricular anatomy, including relationship of the floor of the third ventricle and the basilar artery if considering endoscopic third ventriculostomy (ETV) (see below). It is also the imaging of choice in children to assess the entire neuro-axis in cases of spinal dysraphism and tumour pathology.

Specific treatment

Fontanelle tap

In infants/neonates the anterior fontanelle provides immediate access to the ventricular system to allow reduction in ICP (which can be life-saving if the infant is *in extremis*) and also to allow CSF to be sent for analysis if infection is suspected. 10–20 ml/kg of CSF can be removed by this method, but the acute fluid loss in these infants needs to be replaced ml for ml intravenously.

External ventricular drainage

External ventricular drainage (EVD) allows for a temporary diversion of CSF to an external collection bag. This provides a short-term solution and is used following acute haemorrhage (acute blood will block a shunt) or in the presence of infection. It can also be used to instill intra-thecal drugs (e.g., vancomycin). Usage beyond 10 days increases the risk of ventriculitis.

Shunt placement

Ventricular-peritoneal shunts (pleural and atrial shunts are used less commonly) are the mainstay of hydrocephalus treatment. They allow a permanent diversion of the CSF into the peritoneal cavity. Use of pressure (or flow) valves allows regulation of the amount of CSF that is removed. Lumbo-peritoneal shunts can be used in older children, but only in the presence of a communicating hydrocephalus.

Endoscopic third ventriculostomy

ETV is a newer procedure that is rapidly gaining fashion. The endoscope is used to create a new channel *via* the floor of the third ventricle to allow passage of CSF. Its role is predominantly in the treatment of an obstructive hydrocephalus where the CSF pathway between the third and the fourth ventricle is compromised (e.g., aqueduct stenosis, pineal region and posterior fossa tumours). The endoscope can also be used at the same time to biopsy tumours within the third ventricle/pineal region/aqueduct or to allow introduction of an aqueductal stent.

HEAD INJURY

Children's heads are disproportionately larger than those of adults in relation to their overall body size; this, together with the reliance on ligamentous stability, predisposes them to certain types of brain and cervical spine injury following trauma. Unmyelinated brain has a higher water content than the more developed brain, which makes it softer and more prone to acceleration-deceleration injury. Cerebral water content decreases with age, and thus shear-type forces cause greater harm to the child's brain than is produced by the equivalent force in adults. The presence of an open fontanelle in infants increases their tolerance to raised intracranial pressure in the early stages. A similar 'escape valve' allows slightly older children with open sutures to cope initially with rising pressures. Sutural diastasis is also a common feature in children with fractures. Whereas contre-coup injuries are more commonplace amongst adult head-injured patients, coup injuries are more common in children. The increased compliance of the paediatric cranium leads to direct impaction on the underlying brain following trauma. The scalp is a very vascular region and profuse bleeding can occur from any open wound. It should be remembered that the circulating blood volume in a child is only 80 ml/kg and that haemorrhage from such wounds can lead to hypotension and shock in infants and small children. Similarly, intracranial haemorrhage can be significant enough to cause circulatory distress prior to neurological deficits. Two aspects exclusive to children are in birth and non-accidental injuries (NAI). The presence of a cephalhaematoma or depressed skull fracture may be seen following instrumented delivery. Subdural haematomas may develop in either type of injury. Following birth injury, they can manifest as seizures, pupillary abnormalities or respiratory distress and may develop within a few hours. The presence of a subdural haematoma without any signs of significant trauma or in the absence of a plausible history should raise concerns about NAI.

GOALS OF MANAGEMENT

The goals of management in children with head injury remain no different from those in adults. Primary brain injury occurs at the time of impact and is irreversible. However, further neuronal damage is caused by hypoxia and hypoperfusion. Head injury leads to raised ICP, reduced CPP with loss of autoregulation, and to neuroexcitotoxicity which accentuates these problems. Management should therefore be aimed at preventing secondary brain injury by early treatment of these adverse factors. It is likely that the severely injured child will require standard traumatic resuscitation in accordance with APLS/ATLS guidelines. Airway management with cervical spine control, breathing, and circulatory resuscitation should all be addressed prior to neurological evaluation and specific treatment. In cases of severe injury, management will take place in the paediatric intensive care units (PICU); the underlying basis of management in the 'ward-managed' head-injured children is, however, no different. The goals remain to protect the airway, adequately oxygenate and correct any hypovolaemia and hypotension. The following sections will discuss the rationale behind the management strategies, before considering how patients should be managed on the ward.

AIRWAY AND VENTILATORY MANAGEMENT

In the presence of a severe traumatic brain injury where protection of the airway is essential, urgent consultation with the local PICU team should be sought. The goals of airway management are to provide a safe airway to allow optimization of ventilation, to prevent hypoxaemia, and to maintain normocapnia.

In the past, ventilatory strategies involved prolonged hyperventilation, as this had been shown to decrease ICP, albeit transiently. However, the associated vasoconstriction and decreased cerebral blood flow (CBF) caused more harm from cerebral ischaemia than protection from ICP. In consequence, normocapnia is now the aim, with short transient episodes of hyperventilation used only to treat an 'ICP crisis.' Several studies have shown that hypoxaemia is a significant predictor of morbidity; therefore, maximizing oxygenation is another essential prerequisite. These two factors are equally essential, even in the ward management of those children with a less severe brain injury. Remember the following three principles:

1. *Airway protection*: is the child able to cough and maintain a clear and safe airway? If the child is excessively drowsy consider PICU involvement at an early stage.

2. *Maximize oxygenation*: monitor saturations and give supplemental oxygen as required.

3. *Monitor respiration*: decreased respiratory rates (e.g., drowsiness, opioid drugs) will lead to hypercapnia and increases in ICP. Tachypnoea leads to hypocapnia and the problems addressed above.

CIRCULATORY SUPPORT AND FLUID MANAGEMENT

Cerebral blood flow averages 55–60 ml/100g brain tissue/min in normal adults and is known to be higher in children. It is not known what the critical values of CBF are below which cerebral ischaemia occurs. The most significant factor determining CBF at any time is the cerebral perfusion pressure (CPP). This can be calculated from mean arterial and intracranial pressures (MAP and ICP) by the formula:

$$CPP = MAP - ICP$$

(MAP = 2/3 diastolic pressure + 1/3 systolic pressure).

It therefore follows that maintaining an adequate CPP can be achieved by maintaining an adequate blood pressure, and by reducing any factors that increase ICP. Evidence has shown that improved outcome is inversely proportional to the number of hypotensive episodes, and thus falls in CPP. In the paediatric intensive care unit (PICU) setting, the use of invasive monitoring (arterial and central venous lines) allows for a comprehensive circulatory assessment. Inotropic support can be given to aid falling blood pressure, if required. Again, this important aspect of treatment also requires addressing in ward managed patients. Remember the following principles:

1. *Monitor pulse and blood pressure*: tachycardia may be the first sign of hypovolaemia and needs urgently to be addressed. Has adequate fluid been given during the resuscitative period? Is there another potential bleeding source (e.g., abdominal or long bone injuries)? Bradycardia may be a sign of an expanding intracranial mass lesion but can also be a sign of circulatory failure. Urgent consultation with PICU is again essential.

2. *Check haemoglobin (Hb)*: low Hb values diminish the oxygen-carrying capacity of the blood and may suggest significant blood loss. Circulating blood volume in children is approximately 80 ml/kg and therefore even small losses can lead to significant hypotension.

3. *Keep normovolaemic*: there is an increased risk of hypotensive episodes if the child is kept 'dry'.

4. *Avoid dextrose solutions*: dextrose-containing fluids can lead to a decrease in plasma osmolality and hyponatraemia. This combination leads to an increased osmotic drive into the neuronal cells, leading to increased brain oedema. 0.9% NaCl solutions should be used in preference.

5. *Avoid hyperglycaemia*: hyperglycaemia can also lead to an increase in neural injury (glucose is metabolized to lactic acid and the subsequent fall in tissue pH leads to worsening metabolic injury). Insulin sliding-scale regimens may be required.

INTRACRANIAL PRESSURE MANAGEMENT

Controlling ICP is an important factor in managing patients with head injury. ICP is maintained within normal limits within a reasonable range of increased intracranial volumes. Efflux of CSF and/or venous blood forms a major part of this compensatory mechanism. However, as any intracranial mass lesion expands this compensation is overcome, and a rapid rise in ICP is seen, even with very small increases in intracranial volume. The Monro-Kellie doctrine, proposed in the early part of the 19th century, provides a formula for calculation of intracranial volume and a procedure by which it may be treated.

$$V_{intracranial} = V_{brain} + V_{CSF} + V_{blood} + V_{mass\ lesion}$$

A reduction in any of the four factors on the right-hand side of this equation will lead to a decrease in intracranial volume, and therefore to a drop in ICP. Various methods are available to achieve this, including:

1. *Head up posture*: helps reduce ICP by increasing venous return, reducing V_{blood} and therefore increases CPP. Elevation beyond 30° leads to a more significant decrease in CPP and thus limits the amount of head up recommended.

2. *Early clearance of spinal injury*: cervical collars reduce venous return and can lead to a rise in ICP. In the absence of spinal injury, not only can the collar be removed but the patient can be sat up, which can help ventilation and prevent CO_2 retention.

3. *Drainage of CSF*: insertion of an EVD will allow drainage of CSF, reducing V_{CSF} and thus ICP. Unfortunately, in cases of traumatic brain injury the ventricles are usually small and CSF cannulation may not be possible.

4. *Mannitol*: acts as an osmotic diuretic leading to 'dehydration' of neuronal cells which will decrease V_{brain} and thus reduce ICP. Its effect is short-acting and therefore is best used in the treatment of an ICP 'crisis'.

5. *Sedation/paralysis*: ICU management may involve not only ventilatory support but also medical treatment in reducing ICP. Sedative drugs e.g., propofol, as well as paralytics (e.g., atracurium) reduce pain, agitation and shivering, thereby reducing cerebral metabolic rate (CMR) and thus ICP.

6. *Barbiturate therapy*: these agents are used in the treatment of refractory raised ICP. They are used to induce a barbiturate coma with a view to reducing CMR, cerebral blood volume (CBV) and ICP. They can also act as anticonvulsants.

7. *Surgery*: the presence of an intracranial haematoma (subdural, extradural, contusions) is an indication for surgery if there is significant mass effect or there is evidence of its expanding. It is vital that, prior to surgery, any 'ABC' abnormalities are corrected; in infants and small children, a large intracranial haematoma may cause a significant drop in haemoglobin and may be the predominant cause for the child's critical status.

8. *Seizure management*: neuroexcitotoxicity is not uncommon following head injury and can lead to seizures. This leads to an increase in cerebral metabolic rate and rises in ICP. Post-traumatic seizures are more commonly seen in children than in adults, with up to 10% being affected. The role for prophylactic anticonvulsants in children remains questionable. Studies in adults have shown that prophylactic anticonvulsants reduce the incidence of early seizures (within 1 week), but have no long-term benefit.

Various surgical options are available which include:

1. *ICP monitoring*: insertion of a pressure transducer to monitor ICP can easily be carried out *via* a twist drill procedure. Several transducers are available and can be placed in any of the intracranial compartments, although intraparenchymal monitors are the most commonly used.

2. *EVD placement*: insertion of an EVD can also be performed *via* a (usually right frontal) burrhole. This is only feasible if the ventricles are not effaced, and allows drainage of CSF to help control ICP.

3. *Craniotomy for haematoma*: a standard trauma craniotomy can be used to evacuate a significant extradural, subdural or contusional injury. Burrhole drainage can be used in more chronic haematomas but is not usually indicated in the acute period.

4. *Decompressive craniectomy*: removal of the bone flap to increase the potential space for cerebral swelling (and, in essence, reduce the effect of V_{brain}) remains a controversial area. It is usually reserved for cases when the raised ICP has become refractory and is no longer manageable by medical therapies. At present there is very little evidence that it improves outcome: a single study in Australia suggests there may be a benefit from early decompression in children.

WARD-BASED MANAGEMENT

It is important to obtain a history outlining the nature and severity of the head injury, e.g., height of fall, speed of car, use of seatbelts, etc. This will also give an indication of whether other organs may also have been injured and need addressing. Often, this history has to be obtained from witnesses. The initial cardiorespiratory and neurological condition can best be obtained from members of the paramedic crew (the importance of whom should not be underestimated!). It is important to document the presence of seizures, length of any amnesic periods and any episodes of loss of consciousness. An immunization history, especially a tetanus status, should also be obtained. A full systemic examination is required, especially in cases where it has not been possible to obtain a history. If the preceding history does not support the examination findings consider the possibility of NAI and seek expert help from senior staff and the paediatric service.

General work up

- *U&Es*: vomiting leads to electrolyte imbalance and dehydration.
- *FBC*: even small blood losses in young children can cause significant falls in Hb.
- *Coagulation screen*: risk of disseminated intravascular coagulopathy in trauma patients.
- *Cross-match blood*: at least 2 units.
- *IV cannulation and fluids.*
- *CT scan*: to assess presence of intracranial haematomas, cerebral swelling, midline shift, mass effect, sulcal effacement and bony injuries.

Further Treatment

The majority of ward-based head-injured children can be managed conservatively. It is important to monitor them closely, so that their cardiorespiratory status can be optimized as mentioned above. Adequate analgesia should be provided as pain leads to increases in metabolic rate and also raises ICP. Fever causes a similar reaction and pyrexial events should therefore be investigated early and treated appropriately. Early discussions with PICU should occur in relation to any child in whom there is any cardiorespiratory or neurological compromise. Whilst an expanding mass lesion may be the cause of an acute deterioration, electrolyte imbalances, particularly hyponatraemia, can also lead to neurological dysfunction – don't forget to check the bloods!

PAEDIATRIC BRAIN TUMOURS

Brain tumours are the commonest solid paediatric tumour and comprise 20% of all childhood cancers, being second only in incidence to leukaemia. Although paediatric brain tumours are predominantly infratentorial (approximately 60%), the location of tumours is highly dependent on age. Children under 6 months of age are more likely to have a supratentorial tumour (approximately 75%). The nature of the tumour is also dependent on its location and on the age of the child. Whilst in the infratentorial compartment there is a relatively equal incidence of primitive neuroectodermal tumour (PNET) (most commonly medulloblastoma), brain stem gliomas and pilocytic astrocytomas, in the supratentorial region astrocytomas are significantly more common. Congenital tumours presenting in neonates are more likely to be neuroectodermal in origin, with teratomas being most common, whilst in older children astrocytomas, PNET and ependymomas predominate. Some glial tumours, such as mixed gliomas, are unique to children; they are most frequently located the cerebellum (67%) and are usually benign.

PILOCYTIC ASTROCYTOMA

Juvenile pilocytic astrocytomas occur more often in children and young adults than in older adults. They are the most common astrocytic tumours in children, accounting for 80–85% of cerebellar astrocytomas and 60% of optic gliomas. They comprise about 33% of all posterior fossa tumours in children, and represent about 25% of all paediatric tumours. Juvenile pilocytic astrocytomas usually arise in the cerebellum, brainstem, hypothalamic region, or optic pathways, but they may occur in any area where astrocytes are present, including the cerebral hemispheres and the spinal cord. There is an association with neurofibromatosis: optic nerve gliomas are common tumours in patients with this condition and may present bilaterally. Patients with optic pilocytic astrocytomas associated with neurofibromatosis type 1 (NF1) usually have better outcomes than other patients with juvenile pilocytic astrocytomas.

Pathophysiology

These tumours are usually discrete, indolent lesions associated with cyst formation. The cysts may be unilocular or multilocular, with an associated tumor nodule. The nodular portion of the lesion usually demonstrates homogeneous contrast enhancement. Calcification is present in 10% of juvenile pilocytic astrocytomas. Histologically, the tumour contains fibrillary astrocytes with associated Rosenthal fibers (intracellular, eosinophilic, rod-shaped bodies). The tumour is named after the 'hair-like' bipolar (piloid) astrocytes. Features more typically seen in higher grade gliomas can be seen (nuclear atypia, mitoses, endothelial proliferation, and necrosis), but they have no proven prognostic significance.

Epidemiology

The peak incidence is in patients of 5–14 years of age with no sex predilection.

Treatment

Posterior fossa pilocytic astrocytomas are typically treated with surgery and completely resected whenever possible. Optic nerve tumours can often be managed conservatively and surgery is usually indicated in an attempt to preserve vision in the unaffected eye.

Outcome

Patients with juvenile pilocytic astrocytoma have a better prognosis than do patients with most other types of astrocytomas. If gross total resection is possible, the 10-year survival rate is as high as 90%. After subtotal resection or biopsy, the 10-year survival rate is as high as 45%. Morbidity is related to the location of the tumor and to the associated complications of tumor resection.

PRIMITIVE NEUROECTODERMAL TUMOURS

Primitive neuroectodermal tumours (PNETs) include medulloblastomas, medulloepitheliomas, pigmented medulloblastomas, ependymoblastomas, pineoblastomas, and cerebral neuroblastomas. These tumours originate from undifferentiated cells in the subependymal region in the foetal brain. The frequency of occurrence of PNETs is similar to that of pilocytic astrocytoma. Medulloblastomas initially arise in the inferior medullary velum and grow to fill the fourth ventricle, infiltrating the surrounding structures. They are the most common malignant posterior fossa tumor in the pediatric population. They are characterized by their tendency to seed along the neuro-axis, following CSF pathways, and can rarely metastasize to extraneural tissues. Evidence of 'drop-mets' will be seen in 10–30% of patients at the time of diagnosis. Extra-cranial metastases (involving bone, liver and lymph nodes) account for 5% of cases.

Pathophysiology

Medulloblastomas are highly cellular, vascular tumours with a deeply basophilic nucleus and multiple mitoses ('small blue cell tumour'). These histological features are commonly seen in the other variants of PNET.

Epidemiology

The male : female ratio is approximately 3:1. Medulloblastomas demonstrate a bimodal age distribution with a larger peak occurring at 5–9 years of age, and a smaller peak at 20–30 years of age.

Treatment

Gross surgical excision, followed by craniospinal irradiation, remains the ultimate goal in these patients. However, any attempt to remove tumour from the floor of the fourth ventricle can lead to significant morbidity. Up to 30% of tumours will have invaded the ventricular floor, and care must be taken not to damage this very eloquent region.

Outcome

Children with nondisseminated medulloblastoma, and old enough to have radiation therapy have a 5-year survival rate of about 70%. In the presence of dissemination, adjuvant chemotherapy can be given, but the survival rates are significantly lower. Neurological, endocrine and cognitive deficits are not uncommon in this latter group.

EPENDYMOMA

Ependymomas are derived from ependymal cells and occur most commonly in the ependymal lining of the ventricles. These tumours can also arise in the conus (myxopapillary) and spinal canal. The majority of ependymomas are located in the poterior fossa, with a predilection for the fourth ventricle. Extension through the foramina of Luschka and Magendie is not uncommon. Approximately 10% of patients will have spinal metastases at the time of diagnosis, although this is more common with the anaplastic variants. Tumours presenting supratentorially are more common in adults than in children and are usually located in the trigone of the lateral ventricles.

Pathophysiology

Ependymomas are usually benign tumours which present as solid mass lesions. Histologically, they are composed of uniform ependymal cells forming true rosettes and perivascular pseudo-rosettes. It is not uncommon to have associated calcification, cysts and haemorrhage. Anaplastic ependymomas tend to have histological features of a higher grade tumour with vascular proliferation and necrosis.

Epidemiology

There is a female preponderance with a female:male ratio of approximately 2:1. Median age of presentation is in the second decade but there is a bimodal peak with the younger peak occurring at about age 5 years.

Treatment

Gross total surgical excision where possible, with adjuvant radiotherapy, is the treatment of choice.

Outcome

Combined treatment leads to a 35–60% 5-year survival rate. Although adults have an increased tendency to anaplastic variants, their survival rate is better than children. This is most likely due to the fact that craniospinal radiation therapy is limited to children over the age of 5 years due to the adverse effects on the developing nervous system.

CHOROID PLEXUS PAPILLOMA AND CARCINOMA

Choroid plexus papillomas and carcinomas represent 0.4–0.6% of all intracranial tumours. They represent approximately 3% of childhood brain tumours, and are most likely to occur in the lateral ventricle. Although these tumours can occur in the fourth ventricle, this is a feature that is more commonly seen in adults. Symptoms are usually due to hydrocephalus, which is likely to be due to the presence of increased protein and xanthochromia within the CSF, causing diminished absorption. Overproduction of CSF is not uncommon, but does not explain the persistence of hydrocephalus after tumour removal.

Pathophysiology

Although macroscopically choroid plexus papillomas appear as reddish solid tumours, histologically it can be difficult to differentiate then from normal choroid. As with the other malignant variants of tumour, the presence of nuclear atypia, mitoses and necrosis is suggestive of carcinomatous change.

Epidemiology

Approximately 85% of tumours present in children under 5 years.

Treatment

Surgical resection results in a cure for benign papillomas. These tumours are very vascular and, in the presence of carcinoma, preoperative chemotherapy may have a role in shrinking tumour size and reducing vascularity in order to aid surgical resection.

Outcome

Five-year survival rates of about 80% have been described. The main morbidity arises from persistent subdural collections due to a ventriculo-subdural fistula.

BRAINSTEM GLIOMAS

Overall, brainstem gliomas constitute 15% of all brain tumours. In children, however, brainstem gliomas represent 25–30% of all brain tumours. Most brainstem gliomas are low-grade astrocytomas and can be conservatively managed. Surgical debulking is reserved for exophytic portions of tumour.

Diffuse pontine gliomas are, however, more aggressive (anaplastic astrocytoma or glioblastoma) with a very short survival.

CLINICAL FEATURES OF PAEDIATRIC BRAIN TUMOURS

Mass lesions in children may present in one of three ways: raised ICP; focal neurological signs; and seizures. Pituitary tumours and craniopharyngiomas may present with either neurological deficit (visual loss) or endocrine dysfunction.

MANAGEMENT OF PAEDIATRIC BRAIN TUMOURS

- Remember ABCs!

General work up

- As for hydrocephalus.

Specific work up

- *MRI of brain and spine*: it is preferable to carry out this prior to any surgical intervention, as it is useful to assess suitability for endoscopic managements (e.g., ETV, biopsy) and allows better evaluation of the tumour and its relation to eloquent structures. Furthermore, it allows for assessment of any spinal disease (e.g., drop metastases).

- *Tumour markers*: these are obtainable from CSF and serum; they are essential for optimising management of pineal region tumours.

- *Endocrine assessment*: pituitary and craniopharyngioma patients (may need preoperative hormone replacement).

- *Opthalmology/visual fields*: most commonly required for pituitary patients, but should be assessed in any child with a tumour along the visual pathway.

Treatment options

In most cases, treatment for symptomatic hydrocephalus is carried out first. This has the advantage of rapidly improving symptoms such as headache and vomiting, but also allows investigation of CSF markers. In the presence of an aqueductal stenosis due to an offending tumour, an initial endoscopic approach may be used to create a third ventriculostomy and to biopsy the tumour at the same sitting. Surgical excision is carried out wherever tumour location makes it possible. Unlike in adults, the free use of chemo- and radiotherapy is not possible. Children under the age of 5 years have a significant long-term morbidity with whole brain (+/- spine) radiotherapy. Outcomes are improved in children over 5 years old at diagnosis with no evidence of disseminated disease and maximal surgical resection. Brainstem and optic tract gliomas are usually low-grade astrocytomas, and are predominantly managed conservatively.

Follow-up imaging

MRI within the first 24 h after surgery provides a baseline for further follow-up and for optimizing any adjuvant therapy. The artefact produced from surgical intervention makes radiological assessment of residual tumour after 48 h exceptionally difficult and therefore if imaging cannot be performed within this time period it should be deferred for at least 6 weeks.

10
Basic Neurosurgical Procedures
Reuben D. Johnson

CONTENTS

INTRODUCTION

As a junior neurosurgical trainee you will have the opportunity to see a multitude of complex and dramatic operations. However, you are unlikely to play a large role in them in your early training. In spite of this, some commonly performed procedures may be classified as 'basic' such that junior trainees should be familiar with their principles and performance. They are not minor or easy; rather, they constitute the cases you will repeatedly see on the ward.

This chapter summarizes them, and you should endeavour to see them undertaken early in your post, thus maximising your chance of actually performing at least part of them. Even if your career goal is not neurosurgery, understanding them will be of benefit when managing patients that you refer to or accept from neurosurgery, as you will do in orthopaedics or general surgery.

Neurosurgery involves a significant amount of out of hours operating for potentially life-threatening conditions, often amenable to basic interventions. Specifically: diversion of CSF flow using external ventricular drains (EVDs) and shunts; evacuation of chronic subdural haematomas (CSDH), acute subdural haematomas (ASDH) and extradural haematomas

(EDH); and spinal decompression. These are often the cases that you will manage from admission, and their frequency will provide ample opportunity to familiarize yourself with them.

CRANIAL PROCEDURES

SOME BASIC SURFACE ANATOMY

Opening the cranium requires an appreciation of basic surface anatomy and its relationship to deeper structures. When incising the scalp, appreciation of the location of scalp vessels ensures preservation of scalp flap vascularity. Generally, it is a highly vascular structure, but ideally, to minimize the risk of necrosis, major vessels should not be sacrificed.

There are five arteries, bilaterally, supplying the scalp. Anteriorly are the supratrochlear (medial) and supraorbital (lateral) arteries which arise from the opthalmic branch of the internal carotic artery (ICA). More posteriorly are branches of the external carotid artery: the superficial temporal artery; the posterior auricular artery; and the occipital artery. Plentiful anastamoses exist, but there is a risk of ischaemia unless flaps are based upon one of these arteries. Perhaps the branch most relevant to the junior trainee is the superficial temporal artery, the pulsation of which can be palpated just in front of the tragus. When making the incision for the trauma craniotomy described below, it is prudent to palpate for this artery and begin your incision posterior to it. Another rule to adhere to, is to make sure that the bottom half of the flap is never less than half the length of the top edge.

The nerve supply of the scalp itself is of less concern to the neurosurgeon. However, the temporal branch of the facial nerve can be damaged by an injudiciously placed incision, resulting in a palsy of the frontalis muscle. The temporal branch passes from within the substance of the parotid gland and crosses above the zygomatic arch about 2.5 cm anterior to the tragus; hence incisions in the zygomatic area are kept less than 1¼ cm anterior to the tragus and above the zygomatic arch.

For the purposes of the procedures described here, the next most important structures to be aware of are the dural venous sinuses and the motor strip. Provided that burr-holes are placed well away from these areas, the risks will be kept to a minimum. The sagittal sinus runs in the midline, and so burrs are cut over 2.5 cm from the midline. It is important, when draping patients, to make sure that you can still confidently identify the midline. Other sinuses, such as the lateral sinus, should be well away from your drill, as you should not be cutting near the posterior fossa. The motor cortex is located 4–5 cm behind the coronal suture which, with practice on yourself, should be easily palpable through the scalp. Alternatively, the position of the superior aspect of the motor cortex can be estimated by following a vertical line up through the external auditory meatus. An oft-quoted method is to use a tape measure (or piece of string that can be halved by folding) to find the mid-point of the arc extending from nasion to inion (external occipital protruberance): the motor cortex is 2 cm posterior to this point. Figure 10.1 summarizes these three methods for estimating the position of the motor strip. The transverse sinus can be marked out by drawing a line from the tragus to the external occipital protuberance.

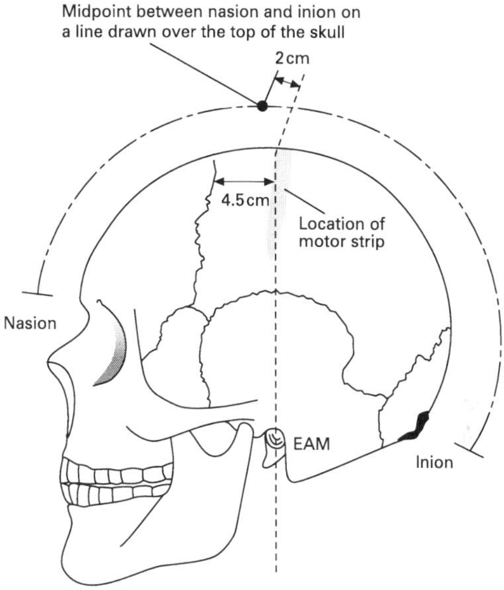

Midpoint between nasion and inion on a line drawn over the top of the skull

2 cm

4.5 cm

Location of motor strip

Nasion

EAM

Inion

Figure 10.1. Diagram summarizing three methods of estimating the position of the motor strip in relation to the skull. EAM = external auditory meatus.

INSERTION OF AN ICP BOLT

Insertion of ICP bolts may be done in the intensive care unit (ICU) to monitor the intracranial pressure (ICP) in patients with diffuse head injury. If a patient goes to theatre, then insertion of ICP-monitoring devices is ideally performed at the time of surgery. If performed in the ICU, it is imperative that the procedure is carried out in as sterile a manner as possible.

Ideally, the surgeon will be positioned at the head of the patient, who is lying supine. Identify, shave, and mark Kocher's point, which is 1 cm anterior to the coronal suture in the midpupillary line, which is about 2.5 cm from the midline (see Figure 10.2). After cleaning the area and injecting some local anaesthetic (e.g., 2 ml lignocaine with adrenaline) make a small vertical stab incision (no more than 0.5 cm long) with a small blade, down to the skull. A twist drill is used to penetrate the skull. There should be a spur or shoulder on the drill to prevent plunging it into the brain. Once the skull has been breached, a small cylindrical tap is screwed into the hole to allow for passage of the ICP catheter (some ICP kits do not have this and the wire is passed directly through the hole). It is advisable to calibrate the ICP monitor at this point before opening the dura. The exact

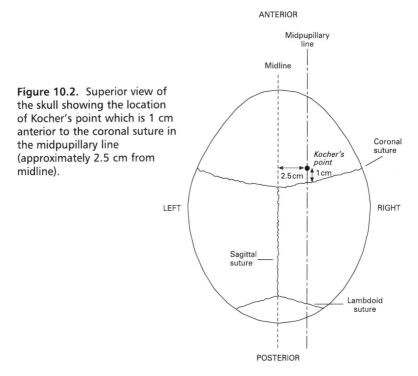

ANTERIOR

Figure 10.2. Superior view of the skull showing the location of Kocher's point which is 1 cm anterior to the coronal suture in the midpupillary line (approximately 2.5 cm from midline).

procedure for calibration will differ between makes of machine, and the ICU staff will usually be familiar with the one they keep in stock (it usually involves obtaining a zero reading whilst the monitor wire is in sterile water, and writing down a reference number). The dura is opened by pricking it with a pin placed down the cylindrical tap. The pin will be provided by the manufacturer and will usually have a right-angle on it to prevent its going too far or being lost inside the cranium. A small back-flow of CSF is usually seen as the pin passes through the dura. The ICP monitor wire can now be passed down the tap (it should not exceed the inner surface of the cranium by more than 0.5 cm) and then screwed securely. Before attaching the ICP monitor wire to the monitor, make sure that it is securely fastened so as to reduce the chances of its being pulled out.

BURR-HOLE DRAINAGE OF A CHRONIC SUBDURAL HAEMATOMA

The drainage of a subdural haematoma can usually be achieved through one or two burr-holes. Two may be helpful, as this allows the washing of saline from one burr-hole through to the next. The location of the burr-holes will depend upon the location of the haematoma as determined by CT scan. However, the general principle is that burr-holes should be located

144

along the same line as the incision of a trauma flap, so that, if there are any problems, it is relatively easy to proceed to a trauma craniotomy. The procedure can be performed under local anaesthetic but until you are more experienced, and unless the patient is likely to tolerate the procedure awake, it is best done under general anaesthetic. The patient is positioned supine on the operating table with the head placed on a ring. Check the side of the haematoma on the scan at this point and double check with a colleague. For burr-holes, the head can be kept straight or slightly angled to the side contralateral to the haematoma. It should be borne in mind that, if it is necessary to proceed to craniotomy, the head will need to be rotated further laterally (see below). Once the head is positioned, the hair can be shaved and the skin incisions marked out (aprox. 2–3 cm in length). The incisions should be placed along the line of an appropriate craniotomy, such as the question-mark-shaped temporoparietal craniotomy described below. Ensure that your incisions are located so that the burr-holes will overlie the subdural haematoma. It is essential, therefore, to look at the scan again and decide the height of the haematoma in the cranium and its anteroposterior extent. Prep and drape the patient so that you can still locate the midline and can feel relevant landmarks, such as the glabella and external auditory meatus. Inform the anaesthetist, and infiltrate local anaesthetic with adrenaline into the sites of your incision. Before picking up the scalpel check the side one more time. If the site of your incision is above the superficial temporal line (which it most probably will be) you will be able to cut directly through skin down to bone. Use the handle of the knife, or the handle of a periosteal elevator, to push the periosteum away from the skull. If you are using two burr-holes, prepare the second site before drilling. Insert a self-retainer to hold the wound open and expose the skull. You will find that the self-retainer will control most bleeding points from the scalp edges, but use bipolar diathermy to control any obvious bleeders.

You are now ready to use the drill. Make sure that you are comfortable and hold the drill in both hands. Make sure that the patient's head is well supported by your assistant. You will be taught how to use the drill, but the following points must always be remembered: apply a constant firm pressure but without leaning your body-weight on the drill; the drill will stop automatically once the cranium is breached and, when it does, take your foot off the drill pedal (and not before, as the clutch will disengage and it will not be possible to start it again.) and withdraw the drill. Never restart the drill in the burr-hole once the drill has stopped. You should now be able to see dura and, if the burr-hole is properly located, you will see the dark blue of the subdural haematoma underneath. Control any bleeding from the bone with bone wax, and remove any fragments of remaining bone with a blunt hook and fine-toothed forceps. Now use the diathermy to scorch the whole area of exposed dura.

Open the dura by making a cruciate incision with an appropriately sized knife and sharp hook. It is safest to make a small incision to begin and then use the hook to lift the dura towards you. Once the dura has been incised in this way there will be four triangular leaves of dura. Shrink these back to the bone by grasping them with the bipolar and coagulating them. If the membranes around the CSDH have not burst by this point then scorch it with the bipolar and open it with a blunt instrument like a Macdonald. Alternatively, hold the bipolar tips close together and advance them into the membrane and allow them to open up (again, scorch the membranes as you advance). Once through, you will find that the dark brown fluid that constitutes a CSDH will drain out. Wash the subdural space through carefully with saline. Some surgeons insert soft catheters into the subdural space to wash it out, but it is important to avoid damage to the brain, and using only a syringe can be a safer option in the junior surgeon's hands. You will see the surface of the brain and you should try to allow it to expand towards the cranium. This may happen spontaneously or you might ask the anaesthetist to induce a Valsalva manoeuvre to speed things up.

Before closing the wounds ensure that you have filled any gaps between the brain and skull as much as possible with saline. You may either leave the burr-holes empty or fill them with Surgicel™, Spongistan™ or beeswax. Close the scalp with 2/0 or 3/0 Vicryl™ interrupted to the galea, and either clips or 3/0 nylon to the skin.

FRONTOTEMPOROPARIETAL TRAUMA CRANIOTOMY
(DRAINAGE OF ASDH AND EDH)

The reason for describing this craniotomy is that the most common site for an ASDH is the surface of the frontotemporoparietal cortex. Also, this incision can be used to evacuate an EDH which has formed in the classic temporal location due to bleeding from the middle meningeal artery.

The patient is positioned supine, with the head rotated to the side contralateral to the clot. The idea is to position the patient in such a way that there will be an optimal view under all edges of the craniotomy. Generally speaking, you should aim to have the side of the head as horizontal as possible. This is facilitated by the placement of sandbags under the ipsilateral shoulder. The head is best fixed with a three-point head fixator.

Shave the side of the head affected, all the way to the midline. Mark out a question-mark-shaped incision which begins at the zygomatic arch no more than a finger's breadth in front of the tragus. Remember to palpate for the superficial temporal artery and avoid it. The line of the incision is a curve back around the top of the ear and then a curve towards the midline. From here it runs parallel to the midline anteriorly to the hairline (see Figure 10.3). Prep and drape the patient.

Make an incision through the scalp along the line described above. This is a large incision and bleeding needs to be adequately controlled. This is achieved by direct pressure either side of the incision with the fingers on mastoid swabs. After every 5 cm or so of incision apply Raney scalp clips

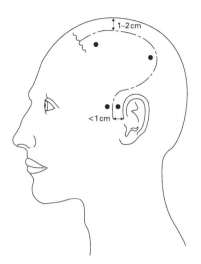

Figure 10.3. Diagram showing the location of a typical skin incision for a frontotemporoparietal craniotomy. Note that the location of four burr-holes is also shown: one frontal; one parietal; and two temporal. It is important to place the two temporal burr-holes low down in order to decompress temporal extradural haematomas.

over the scalp edges to include the mastoid swabs. This should be an efficient, smooth process so as not to delay proceeding to the life-saving part of the operation. Part of your incision may take you directly down to bone, but in the temporal area it will overlie the temporalis muscle. You will need to sweep the scalp forward over the surface of the muscle using a wet swab and the back of the scalpel blade to expose the muscle. Wrap the scalp flap in a wet swab and anchor it forward out of the way with rubber bands.

Cut through the temporalis muscle down to bone with the monopolar diathermy. The line of incision is just inside your skin incision in an inverted 'U' shape. Remember that, when you come to use the craniotome, you need to be about 3 cm from the midline so as to stay away from the sagittal sinus. Leave the lowermost neck of temporalis intact. Sweep the periosteum clear with the periosteal elevators along the line of the incision.

Place four burr-holes: one temporal; one at the pterion; one frontal; and one parietal. Connect the burr-holes with the craniotome. Use bone elevators to lift the bone flap gently away from the dura, taking care not to tear the dura as you do so. You are now left with either of two situations, depending on the indication for the operation. You will see either a bright red EDH overlying the dura or a dark blue ASDH underneath the dura.

In the case of an EDH, you have already performed the life-saving procedure by opening the bone. There remains only to evacuate the haematoma by sucking away at it, and then placing dural hitch stitches to attach the dura to the edges of the craniotomy. This is to prevent the EDH from reaccumulating. Use a non-cutting needle and 3/0 Vicryl™, taking care not to tear the dura or cause subdural bleeding by making sure that the needle passes only through the outer layer of the dura. It can be useful to slip a single layer of Surgicel™ between the dura and the bone to help haemostasis.

When sucking away the haematoma, identify and control any bleeding points. Look under the edges of the craniotomy and remove any clots found. In the case of a subdural haematoma it is necessary to incise the dura to evacuate the underlying clot. Beware opening the dura too widely as the brain may swell and herniate out of your incision, risking laceration on the sharp dural edges. This is true for cases where it is obvious from the CT scan that there is a lot of brain swelling and mass effect from the haematoma, and in these cases it is safer simply to fenestrate the dura with small slit lacerations and suck out the clot gently. This allows clot evacuation while minimizing brain herniation.

The bone flap can be replaced and either fixed back with screws or bioplates, or allowed to ride free. Riding free may help control the ICP postoperatively. The scalp is closed with 2/0 or 3/0 Vicryl™ to the galea, and clips to the skin. This is a large flap and so a drain may be needed. When removing the Raney's ensure that you take care to diathermy any bleeding points as there can be profuse bleeding at this stage.

In the very acute situation, especially with an EDH, only the lower part of this exposure need be used. For example, in the case of a temporal EDH the first 5 cm or so of the incision can be made and the temporalis incised down to bone. A self-retainer is inserted and a temporal burr-hole made. This can be enlarged quickly using bone-clippers or rongeurs. This allows for extremely rapid decompression of the clot and can be life-saving.

INSERTION OF AN EXTRAVENTRICULAR DRAIN

Insertion of a catheter into the frontal horn of the lateral ventricle is a life-saving procedure in acute hydrocephalus, and familiarity with the technique is essential. The patient is positioned supine with the head secured either on a ring or with a foam cushion. If the head is kept in the neutral position it is easier to coordinate catheter trajectory later on. Shave the right frontal area (the nondominant side is usual for catheter placement, unless there is a contraindication, e.g., underlying lesion). Identify and mark Kocher's point which is 1 cm anterior to the coronal suture in the midpupillary line (approximately 2.5 cm from midline). This is the point at which the burr-hole will be made and the catheter inserted. Mark out a 2–3 cm incision centred on this point in a sagittal plane. Incise the scalp and fashion a burr-hole as described above. In this instance the dura does not need to be opened widely but just sufficiently to allow passage of the catheter. Scorch the pial covering of the cortex with the bipolar diathermy and use the tip of a sharp blade to ensure that it has been breached.

The next step is the most difficult part – placement of the catheter into the frontal horn of the lateral ventricle. There are numerous stereotactic methods described in the books and each is slightly different. The key is to have one method in mind, learn it and stick to it. Basically, if you pass the catheter perpendicular to the surface of the skull to a depth of 5 cm (less in the presence of hydrocephalus) you will enter the frontal horn of the lateral ventricle. There are 5 cm and 10 cm markings on ventricular catheters. To help you ensure that the catheter is perpendicular you can check your position in the coronal and sagittal planes. In the coronal plane the catheter should be pointing towards the medial canthal line of the ipsilateral eye. In the sagittal plane the catheter should be pointing towards the external auditory meatus, or just anterior to it. When the catheter enters the ventricle you should feel a subtle 'give' and when the trocar is withdrawn you will drain CSF. Now advance the catheter with the trocar withdrawn. At this point it is imperative not to let the catheter move in relation to the skull. Hold the catheter with a pair of non-toothed forceps held flush to the skull while you tunnel the distal end of the catheter under the scalp to an exit point a few centimetres away from the skin wound. You would be well advised to secure the catheter in place with a few overlying sutures before closing the scalp incision. Attach your extraventricular drainage system and set it to a fixed setting, e.g., 10 cm H$_2$O.

Close the scalp incision, taking care not to perforate the drain with your needle. Ensure that you secure the drain with a further series of sutures, as EVDs have a tendency to 'fall out' when patients are transferred.

INSERTION OF A VENTRICULOPERITONEAL SHUNT (OCCIPTAL CATHETER)

The patient is supine with a sandbag under the ipsilateral shoulder to allow good rotation of the head away from the site of insertion. The aim is to position the patient so as to provide as straight a line as possible from the occipital site of insertion distally across the neck and thorax to the abdominal site of insertion. Mark out the following: (1) the site of the occipital burr-hole (6 cm superior to the external occipital protruberance and 3 cm from the midline); (2) an incision around the burr-hole so that the incision does not lie over the top of the shunt site; (3) an abdominal incision. Prep the whole area all the way from head to abdomen. Drape to expose the whole shunt path. It may be necessary to staple drapes in the neck area to ensure that they are flush with the skin. Stop, and go through in your mind the sequence of events:

1. Open scalp and drill burr-hole – do not open dura.
2. Open abdomen – clip, but do not open peritoneum.
3. Tunnel, and pass distal catheter (and valve, if attached to catheter).
4. Open dura and pass proximal catheter.
5. Connect proximal catheter to valve (in the case of separate shunt-valve kits).
6. Check CSF flow through shunt.
7. Open peritoneum and pass distal catheter.
8. Close wounds.

Before proceeding, prepare the shunt by taking it out of its packaging and priming and soaking it in gentamicin. Make a curved scalp incision around the planned site of the burr-hole. The site of the burrhole is 6 cm up from the inion (external occipital protruberance) and 3 cm lateral to the midline. Take great care with haemostasis at this stage (you can use monopolar once you are through the skin if you prefer). It is useful to have forceps and mastoid swabs in one hand and diathermy in the other. Remember that water runs down-hill, so start at the top of the wound and work down, otherwise your view will always be obscured by bleeders higher up. Also, cut vessels have two ends, so always check the other side of the wound if you find a big bleeder on one side. A useful tip is to develop scalp layers so that the aponeurosis can be separated and flipped back. This can be sutured over the proximal catheter later, adding strength to the proximal catheter.

Use scissors to develop a plane distally for receipt of valve and catheter: place the scissors in closed, then open them up and withdraw. Make the burr-hole. Cover the proximal wound with Betadine™-soaked swabs. Take care never to touch the edges of wounds.

Now go to the abdomen and open it up. This is similar to an appendix incision, except that it is in the upper part of the abdomen: knife to skin; Langenbecks through fat; scissors through muscle; clips to peritoneum (do not open yet). Leave the clips on the peritoneum and cover the wound with Betadine™-soaked swabs.

You are now ready to tunnel and pass the distal shunt. It is advisable to change gloves at this stage. Place clean swabs over the abdomen so that the shunt end can remain as sterile as possible once passed. It is academic whether you tunnel in a distal-to-proximal direction or *vice versa*. Bend the guide to the correct shape first (use the surface of the patient as a guide). Take care to advance over the clavicle and not to burrow into the neck. Remove the central trocar and pass the shunt through.

Now open the dura with diathermy in the centre of the burr-hole and pass the tip of the knife through. Use diathermy to extend the hole slightly and then buzz the surface of the brain only slightly. Pass the proximal catheter directed towards the glabella to a depth of 4 cm (or check the distance on the scan) and feel for entry into the ventricle. Remove the trocar to check for CSF flow and advance the catheter. Place the bulldog clip on the catheter to control the CSF flow and cut the catheter to the length required (i.e., almost flush with the skull – be careful not to lose the proximal catheter inside the cranium at this stage!).

Connect the two parts of the shunt system and tie securely with 2/0 Vicryl™. Take care not to pull the proximal catheter out at this stage. Remove the bulldog clip and check for CSF flow distally; aspirate if necessary.

Close the head wound with 2/0 or 3/0 Vicryl™ and clips to skin (it is best to use clips, as needles risk perforating the shunt). Remember that, if you developed the scalp layers, the aponeurosis can be flapped over the proximal catheter for extra protection.

Open the peritoneum by holding up the attached clips and checking with thumb and forefinger for the bowel before opening with the scissors. Introduce the distal end of the shunt into the peritoneal cavity. There is no need to suture the peritoneum unless you have made more than a very tiny incision. Close the aponeuroses and muscle with 3/0 Vicryl™ and use subcutaneous Vicryl™ to skin.

SPINAL PROCEDURES

LUMBAR PUNCTURE

The patient is positioned on their side with their knees curled up towards the chest. The back, straight or flexed anteriorly, should be close to the edge of the bed. As the spinal cord ends at L1/2 (continuing as the cauda equina below) the ideal intervertebral space to aim for is L4/5. This can be identified easily, as the highest point of the iliac crest is located on a level with the spinous process of the fourth lumbar vertebra. Feel for the space between the L4 and L5 spinous processes and mark the spot. It is helpful to ensure that, when the area has been cleaned and draped, it is possible to feel the iliac crest without contaminating the hands: this allows the level to be rechecked. Local anaesthetic is injected down to bone and below the skin. The spinal needle is advanced slowly in the midline in the L4/5 interspace in a slightly rostral orientation. The needle will be felt to 'give' when the dura is breached, and a backflash of CSF will be seen when the trocar is withdrawn. The central trocar should now be removed and a manometer attached to measure the opening pressure (this should always be done). A three-way tap attached between the manometer and spinal needle will allow CSF from the manometer to be taken for analysis. If the L4/5 interspace is not encountered the first time then further attempts can be made with the same needle, provided that the tip is not withdrawn from the skin between passes. Always make sure that the patient is as comfortable as possible, and enquire expressly about nerve root pain in the legs (withdraw the needle if pain is felt).

LUMBAR DRAIN PLACEMENT

The procedure to place a lumbar drain is similar to that for a lumbar puncture, except that a larger needle is used which has an angled opening at the tip. This allows a drain to be inserted and guided into the vertebral canal. Care should be taken to orientate the bevel so that the sharp cutting-edge runs parallel to the nerve roots. This reduces the risk of severing the root on insertion. Once in the canal, the needle can be rotated 90° to direct the passage of the drain into the canal.

LAMINECTOMY

The most common laminectomies that are encountered are lumbar and cervical, although thoracic laminectomies will also be seen. The positioning and techniques will differ for each, but the basic principles are the same for all three regions. Patients undergoing cervical laminectomy will be prone, and their heads will be fixed firmly, e.g., with a Mayfield; this is described as the Concorde position, as the neck is in flexion. It is important to ensure that the face of the patient is not pressing on anything that may cause injury, and that the anaesthetist is happy with the airway. In patients undergoing lumbar laminectomy it is important to ensure that the abdomen is not under any pressure, as this would result in increased venous pressure and excessive bleeding in the surgical field. Pressure can be reduced with the use of a pillow under the pelvis and one higher up at the level of the thorax.

There are several ways of determining the spinal level for the laminectomy. One way is to use spinal needles and the image intensifier. However, it may be better to prep and drape the patient beforehand to minimize the risk of infection. Once the levels have been marked, an appropriate midline incision can be marked out. After infiltration of local anaesthetic, a midline incision is made down to the spinous processes. If the incision is truly in the midline then there will be minimal damage to the paravertebral muscles.

The muscles are detached from the spinous processes with cutting diathermy. Care should be taken at the depths of the wound to ensure that the diathermy is not pushed through the interspinous spaces into the spinal canal. The muscle is then stripped away from the laminae with a retractor and mastoid swabs. The rectangular mastoids are inserted vertically into the wound parallel to the spinous processes. The cob is then used to sweep the mastoids laterally out along the laminae, thus lifting the paravertebral muscles away from the bone. A self-retaining retractor system can now be used to hold the wound open. The spinous processes and the laminae should now be clearly visible. It may be necessary to take some time to clean any remaining tissue from the bone. The spinal level should be checked again at this point, using artery clips as markers and visualising with the image intensifier.

The relevant spinous processes are removed by using a Leksell bone rongeurs to break them away from the laminae. The Horsley's can be used in 'Herring bone' fashion to remove the remaining bases of the spinous processes.

The ligamentum flavum is breached with a blunt impliment to enter the spinal canal and the opening is extended using a 1–2 mm Kerrison punch carefully placed under the edge of the laminae. The first bites should be done with caution and the punch should never be forced into a space. If there is any doubt, probe carefully again with a blunt instrument. With diligence and persistence an opening will eventually be made and the spinal canal can be opened. The opening can be increased gradually by taking bites from alternate sides and working up the canal (using a larger 3–5 mm punch, provided that it fits). Care must be taken not to puncture the dura or to take bites out of the nerve roots. As a general rule, work upwards when removing bone and downwards when removing ligamentum. Knowledge of the anatomy of the spinal cord and vertebral canal is essential for this to be done safely. Remember: unless the surgeon knows which parts of the procedure are risky, it is not safe to proceed.

The canal is opened over a given number of predetermined vertebral levels. If the procedure is for decompression of a stenosis, then the canal is widened until the dura is free and not compressed. Otherwise the canal is opened only so far as is required, e.g., for the removal of an extradural abscess or tumour.

The wound is closed with several layers of deep Vicryl™ suture. The surgeon's preference will determine the skin suture.

11
Hydrocephalus and Shunt Systems

Hammad Qureshi, Deb Roy and Reuben Johnson

CONTENTS

INTRODUCTION

Hydrocephalus is a condition in which there is abnormal enlargement of the ventricles due to an excessive accumulation of cerebrospinal fluid (CSF) resulting from a disturbance of its flow, absorption or – less commonly – secretion. Hydrocephalus occurs in approximately 1 per 1000 live births; the incidence of adult onset hydrocephalus is unknown. Hydrocephalus in the paediatric age group is discussed in Chapter 9.

Details of the pathological basis of hydrocephalus are given in Chapter 3 and are recapitulated here as a prelude to the discussion of shunt systems.

CSF PHYSIOLOGY

The predominant site of CSF production is the choroid plexus. A small proportion may be produced by the ependyma and brain parenchyma. CSF is produced at a rate of about 0.4 ml/min (i.e., in the region of 500 ml/day) in an average adult. The total volume of CSF varies with age: in the adult it is 100–150 ml, out of which 15–25 ml are contained within the ventricular system.

CSF flows from the lateral ventricles through the foramina of Munro into the 3rd ventricle and then *via* the aqueduct of Sylvius into the 4th ventricle. From the 4th ventricle it then flows through the foramina of Lushka and Magendie into the basal cisterns and the subarachanoid space. CSF bathes the basal cisterns and the spinal subarachnoid space and then flows over the cerebral hemispheres. It is largely absorbed by the arachnoid villi of the dural sinuses.

CLASSIFICATION OF HYDROCEPHALUS

There are a number of ways to classify hydrocephalus. However, the most useful classification system is the dichotomous one of obstructive (non-communicating) *versus* communicating hydrocephalus.

OBSTRUCTIVE HYDROCEPHALUS

This is caused by an obstruction, due either to external compression or to intraventricular mass lesions, ultimately preventing the CSF from flowing into the subarachnoid space. Dilatation of the ventricular system occurs proximal to the site of obstruction.

- Foramen of Monro obstruction may lead to dilatation of one or, if the obstruction is large enough (e.g., in colloid cyst), both lateral ventricles.
- The aqueduct of Sylvius may be obstructed by a number of genetic or acquired lesions (e.g., atresia, ependymitis, haemorrhage or tumour) and lead to dilatation of both lateral ventricles as well as of the third ventricle.
- Fourth ventricle obstruction (e.g., by a posterior fossa tumour) will lead to a dilatation of the aqueduct as well as of the lateral and third ventricles
- The foramina of Luschka and foramen of Magendie may be obstructed due to congenital failure of opening (e.g., Dandy-Walker malformation).

Congenital hydrocephalus is usually of the obstructive type (see Chapter 9). Consult Chapter 5, on the interpretation of CT head scans, and look particularly at Figures 5.10, 5.12, 5.13, 5.14, 5.20 and 5.22, which show features associated with obstructive hydrocephalus.

Generally speaking, lumbar puncture is contraindicated in obstructive hydrocephalus. It is therefore essential to seek senior advice if lumbar puncture is to be considered.

COMMUNICATING HYDROCEPHALUS

This is caused by impaired CSF reabsorption in the absence of any obstruction of CSF flow between the ventricles and subarachnoid space. It has been postulated that this is due to functional impairment of the arachnoid granulations, which are located along the superior sagittal sinus. Various neurological conditions may result in communicating hydrocephalus; these include subarachnoid/intraventricular haemorrhage, meningitis, Chiari malformation, and congenital absence of arachnoid granulations. Scarring and fibrosis of the subarachnoid space, following infectious, inflammatory, or haemorrhagic events, can also prevent reabsorption of CSF, causing diffuse ventricular dilatation.

Rarely, communicating hydrocephalus is caused by oversecretion of CSF, as in the case of choroid plexus papilloma.

CLINICAL FEATURES

The major presenting features of hydrocephalus are due to signs and symptoms of raised intracranial pressure, i.e., headache, vomiting, papilloedema and deterioration of conscious state. Upgaze is often impaired due to pressure of the dilated 3rd ventricle on the superior colliculus of the tectum. Hydrocephalus may also present as slowly progressive deterioration in the form of headaches, failing mental function, memory loss and behavioural disturbances.

The most important investigation is either computerized tomography (CT) or magnetic resonance imaging (MRI) of the brain. A contrast CT scan or MRI will help determine the cause of hydrocephalus. Where indicated, lumbar puncture confirms high CSF pressure. An intracranial pressure (ICP) monitor may be useful to record CSF pressures over a period of time.

It is important to discuss the following entities which a basic surgical trainee is likely encounter during his/her period of training in neurosurgery.

NORMAL PRESSURE HYDROCEPHALUS

Normal pressure hydrocephalus (NPH) was first described as a clinical entity by Hakim and Adams in 1965. They described a group of elderly patients with a classic triad of dementia, ataxia and incontinence, in whom radiological studies showed hydrocephalus even though lumbar CSF pressure was normal.

Although lumbar pressure is, by definition, normal in patients with NPH, continuous ICP monitoring in these patients will nevertheless reveal abnormal wave formation, especially at night. Some centres routinely perform a CSF infusion study *via* lumbar puncture to estimate the values of various parameters, including CSF outflow resistance. This helps to predict the group of patients who would benefit from a ventriculoperitoneal (VP) shunt procedure.

Another term to remember is hydrocephalus *ex vacuo*, which refers to enlargement of the cerebral ventricles and subarachnoid spaces. This is usually due to brain atrophy (as it occurs in dementias with small vessel ischaemia), post-traumatic brain injuries, and even in some psychiatric disorders, such as schizophrenia. As opposed to hydrocephalus, this is a compensatory enlargement of the CSF-spaces in response to brain parenchyma loss – it is not the result of increased CSF pressure.

IDIOPATHIC INTRACRANIAL HYPERTENSION

Idiopathic intracranial hypertension (IIH), also known as benign intracranial hypertension (BIH) or pseudotumour cerebri (PTC), is a neurological disorder characterized by an increased intracranial pressure in the absence of ventriculomegaly, intracranial mass, infection or hypertensive encephalopathy. This is a diagnosis of exclusion. Some authorities also exclude patients with dural sinus thrombosis.

Most patients with IIH are young, obese females. The peak incidence is in the third decade. The main symptoms are headache, nausea and vomiting, as well as visual symptoms including visual field loss. If untreated, IIH can progress to blindness. This condition is associated with menstrual irregularities or with taking the oral contraceptive pill. An endocrine disturbance has been suggested, but careful studies have failed to show significant endocrine abnormalities.

The diagnosis of IIH is confirmed by demonstrating raised CSF pressures on lumbar puncture and demonstrating a decrease in symptoms following drainage of 30–50 ml of CSF. Most patients are managed medically with weight loss and diuretics, e.g., acetazolamide. The visual symptoms can sometimes be alleviated by optic nerve fenestrations done by ophthalmologists. It is essential to image the venous dural sinuses (e.g., using MR venography) to rule out the presence of venous sinus obstruction which may require a sinus stenting procedure by interventional neuroradiologists. In some patients, a CSF diversion procedure in the form of lumboperitoneal shunt or VP shunt is necessary.

TREATMENT OF HYDROCEPHALUS
HISTORICAL BACKGROUND

The treatment of hydrocephalus has a long history. It was treated surgically even in the time of Hippocrates (460–370 BC) who described the use of trepination and 'lemnisci' (bands of bark which were twisted around the skull and inserted into the trepanned openings in the skull). Vesalius gave the first full description of hydrocephalus in post-renaissance Europe, and observed that, in the adult, hydrocephalus could occur without any external signs. Robert Whytt (1714–1766) is credited with giving the first full description of hydrocephalus as a disease entity; he experimented with numerous pharmacological remedies without success. Alexander Munro (Secundus) (1733–1817) described the use of a lance to puncture the ventricle directly: it is thought likely that this was a treatment already in practice at the time. Subsequently, prominent neurologists and neurological surgeons, including Carl Wernicke (1848–1905) and William Keen (1837–1932), also turned their attention to the treatment of hydrocephalus by external drainage of CSF. Possibly the first account of the diversion of CSF to another location within the body was given by Johann von Mikulicz (1850–1905) who described the use of nail-shaped glass wool which passed from the ventricles to the subgalea. Cushing described the use of lumbar-peritoneal CSF diversion, and Dandy performed a third ventriculostomy in 1920. It was, however, the development of the Spitz-Holter valve, in 1955, which led to the popularization of ventriculoperitoneal shunting.

The treatment of hydrocephalus has, therefore, progressed from external CSF drainage to internal CSF diversion, with or without a shunt system, and almost every body cavity and space has been utilized to absorb the diverted CSF. Modern shunt systems are designed to optimize the process of CSF diversion whilst minimizing the risks of complications of these procedures.

TREATMENT STRATEGIES

Acute deterioration

In acutely deteriorating hydrocephalus, the treatment procedures include:

- External ventricular drain (EVD)
- Lumbar puncture (communicating hydrocephalus)
- Endoscopic third ventriculostomy (obstructive hydrocephalus)
- Ventriculoperitoneal shunt

Gradual deterioration:

When deterioration is gradual, treatment is by means of the following procedures

- Ventriculoperitoneal shunt
- Lumboperitoneal shunt

TYPES OF SHUNT

The three main categories of shunt are:

- Ventriculoperitoneal (most commonly used)
- Ventriculoatrial
- Lumboperitoneal

Apart from the peritoneum or right atrium, distal catheters can also be placed in the pleural cavity and rarely in the gall bladder, ureter or urinary bladder.

COMPONENTS OF A SHUNT

There are four components of a shunt: the proximal catheter; the reservoir; the valve; and the distal catheter.

- Ventricular/lumbar catheter
- Reservoir (permits CSF aspiration for analysis)
- Valve
  a. fixed pressure (Heyer-Shulte, Hakim);
  b. flow regulated (with antisiphon device, e.g., Delta, Orbis, Sigma);
  c. programmable (e.g., Medos, Sophy). The advantage of this type of valve is that the settings can be changed noninvasively following shunt procedure; it is important to note that settings may spontaneously alter following MRI magnetic exposure.
- Distal catheter

SHUNT TECHNIQUE

Shunt surgery requires meticulous attention to detail. Preoperatively, patients should have routine bloods including coagulation screen and group-and-save. Shunts should be performed in daylight hours, if possible, with a minimum number of staff in the theatre and masks worn by all. It is advisable to handle shunts with instruments and not hands, and contact between shunt and skin should be prevented. Antibiotics at the time of shunt induction are strongly recommended. Haemostasis should be addressed with great care throughout the procedure.

Position

Under general anaesthesia, the head is rotated to the side opposite the shunt placement, and the neck extended so that there is almost a straight line between scalp and abdominal incisions. A sandbag under the ipsilateral shoulder allows good rotation of the head to the other side.

Hair is clipped in the operating theatre. Mark the sites of (a) burr hole and the curved incision around it, and (b) the abdominal incision.

Burr hole sites
Posterior parietal approach
The burr hole is located at Keen's Point for a posterior parietal approach – 3 cm posterior and 3 cm superior to the pinna.

Frontal approach
Kocher's point is used for a frontal approach – 3 cm from the midline and 1 cm anterior to the coronal suture in the mid–pupillary line. This is particularly helpful if neck rotation is restricted and parieto-occipital exposure is diffcult.

Occipital approach
For an occipital approach, the burr hole is located on the flat of the occiput, 3–4 cm from the midline along the course of the lamdoid suture.

Shunt induction
The skin is meticulously prepped from the head to the abdomen and adhesive drapes are used to cover the patient such that the whole of the shunt path is exposed. At this stage, prepare the shunt by removing it from its packaging. It is an option to secure the valve to the proximal end of the distal catheter at this stage. The shunt system is primed and left to soak in gentamicin solution.

A small scalp incision is adequate, and a pocket for the valve must be created distal to the scalp incision. A burr hole is made using a perforator or twist drill. The dura is not opened at this stage, and the wound left covered by a betadine-soaked swab.

The abdominal incision may be sited as vertical upper midline, transverse paraumbilical or subcostal. The abdomen is opened in layers, and one has to be definite that the peritoneum is truly opened, with clips left on the peritoneum for identification. Some apply a purse string suture to the peritoneum to prevent the omentum from herniating. Again the wound is covered with a betadine-soaked swab.

It is advisable to change gloves before tunnelling. Care must be taken while tunnelling, especially over the clavicle. If the tunneller goes too deep, injury can be caused to neck structures, or potentially the chest can be entered! If tunnelling is too superficial, skin laceration can occur. Once tunnelling has been completed, the trocar is removed and tubing is passed through.

The dura is now opened and a ventricular catheter is used to cannulate the ventricle. The ventricular catheter trajectory is determined according to external landmarks and available imaging. The ventricular catheter can usually be felt to pop once the ependyma has been breached, and there is a gush of CSF.

The system should be connected to the valve using a tie and the valve tucked into the pocket that has been created; the shunt system is then secured to the pericranium. Ensure that there is CSF flow distally before placing the tube in the peritoneal cavity.

Scalp and abdominal wounds are closed in layers with meticulous attention paid to haemostasis.

See Chapter 10 for further discussion of the insertion of a ventriculoperitoneal shunt using the occipital approach.

Complications

The main complications of shunt placement are:

- *Infection*. Ventriculitis, meningitis, peritonitis or inflammation along the subcutaneous channel. In patients with a ventriculoatrial (VA) shunt, bacteraemia may lead to shunt nephritis. *Staphylococcus epidermidis* or *Staphylococcus aureus* are usually involved. If there is established infection, removal of the shunt is advisable and treatment instituted with antibiotics as per microbiology advice.

- *Subdural haematoma due to shunt overdrainage.*

- *Low pressure state*. Headache and vomiting while sitting or standing. This requires rehydration and gentle mobilization. If this is not adequate, insertion of an anti-siphon device or conversion to a high pressure valve is required.

- *Shunt obstruction*. A shunt system blocked with choroid plexus, debris, omentum or blood clot, results in intermittent or persistent recurrence of symptoms.

- *Bleeding*. (e.g., intraparenchymal or intraventricular). There is the potential for this to happen anywhere along the shunt path.

- *Intra abdominal complications*. (e.g., bowel obstruction, bowel or viscus injury). This can happen during the operation; occasionally, peritoneal tubing can cause erosion into bowel or viscus at a later stage.

- *Other complications*. These include shunt fracture, displacement, seizures (rare) and risks from general anaesthesia.

Further discussions of the causes of shunt system failure, and of the ways in which these problems may be managed, are to be found in Chapters 3 and 7.

12
Neuronavigation and Intra-Operative Imaging
Julian Woollard and Reuben D. Johnson

CONTENTS

INTRODUCTION

One of the fundamental challenges facing a neurosurgeon is the accurate localization of a target, both intracranially and in the spine. The combination of technical skill, imaging, and sound anatomical knowledge enables the neurosurgeon to navigate to a specific area in the CNS. This must be achieved with minimal access and damage to surrounding healthy tissue. Throughout the history of the specialty, different techniques and technologies have been developed to this end.

Aids to neuronavigation can be divided broadly into those which help identify a gross structural location, such as computerized tomography (CT) and magnetic reasonance imaging (MRI), and others which map out a functional area of the brain, such as functional MRI (fMRI), positron emission tomography (PET) and electroencephalography (EEG).

HISTORICAL BACKGROUND

The most basic form of navigation uses surface anatomy of the skull and its relationship to areas of the brain. For example, the motor cortex is situated approximately 4.5 cm posterior to the coronal suture. There is inter-patient variation, and there are obvious inaccuracies to this method, but it serves as a fairly consistent orientation tool. Improvements to this method came with the introduction of plain film radiographs of the skull. Air could be introduced into the ventricles in a pneumoencephalogram, delineating some basic intracranial landmarks for the operating surgeon to navigate by. This was improved further by the introduction of contrast medium into the ventricles. Any effacement of the ventricular system would reveal evidence of mass effect and allude to tumour location. Measurements could be made on preoperative images and correlated with palpable anatomical landmarks to guide craniotomy site and brain dissection.

The advent of CT and the MRI was a huge step forward in terms of target localization and navigation in the CNS, enabling accurate measurements to be made in three planes orthogonal to each other: coronal, sagittal and axial. Modern neuronavigation uses the principles of stereotaxy, where the use of the Cartesian coordinate system enables any point in the brain to be specified by measuring distances along these three intersecting planes. More recently, sophisticated image integration systems have been developed to guide the surgeon more accurately to a particular target.

STEREOTAXY

Stereotaxic surgery involves the use of an external frame fixed to the patient's skull using pins. Once imaged, the frame provides reference points for the calculation of coordinates to any given location within the cranium. The coordinates are distances in each of the three-dimensional (3-D) planes. Using these coordinates, a trajectory can be determined and plotted from the frame to the target, allowing the introduction of surgical instruments to be done accurately. The CT images taken of a patient with the stereotactic frame in place can be fused with preoperative MR images to aid in the localization of deep brain targets. This form of surgery has experienced a revival in the last 15 years due in part to its suitability for the placement of electrodes used to stimulate deep brain nuclei in the management of Parkinson's disease, dystonia, essential tremor, chronic pain syndromes, and some forms of epilepsy. Stereotactic surgery is also used for accurate and minimally invasive brain biopsy.

This technique also has its drawbacks, namely its accuracy and the size of its target. It cannot be used for tumour resection, which requires a wider operative field. This has led to the development of frameless stereotaxy, which relies on the integration of preoperatively acquired CT or MRI data with patient reference points. These can either be anatomical or topically applied fiducial points. The transformed data set allows the guidance of surgical instruments within a three-dimensional coordinate system, which integrates preoperative 'virtual world' images and 'real world' patient anatomy.

For intracranial mass lesions, such as primary or secondary tumours, the boundary between normal and diseased tissue can be very ill-defined. Even when an intracranial mass lesion is discrete from the surrounding brain, optimal planning of the surgical approach is paramount for carrying out a safe excision with minimal damage to healthy tissue. Although still a matter of controversy, there is increasing evidence to suggest that, at least in low-grade gliomas, length of survival is related to degree of resection, with longer-term survival being associated with a greater degree of resection. Throughout an operation using frameless stereotactic guidance, the surgeon can identify a point on the patient and visualise the anatomical location of that same point on a screen showing the preoperative CT/MRI. This enables greater accuracy of resection to the margins of diseased tissue.

Both of these stereotactic techniques rely on a stable relationship between the skull and brain. Inaccuracy can develop due to dynamic changes during surgery known as 'brain shift' within the cranium. This may occur with the release of CSF after dural opening, or after the evacuation of diseased tissue and its associated mass effect. This problem, along with the pursuit of complete tumour resection, has prompted the development of intra-operative imaging.

INTRA-OPERATIVE IMAGING

Neurosurgical units providing intra-operative MRI have shown the value of the procedure in increasing the extent of tumour resection. This emerging navigation modality is likely to become of particular value in cases where maximal tumour resection is paramount, for example paediatric tumours. Currently, its availability is limited due to cost and the requirement for non-ferromagnetic surgical instruments.

Although a rapidly advancing technology, intra-operative CT is only just beginning to reach adequate spatial resolution for applications with intracranial surgery. It is, however, particularly useful for spinal surgery, guiding the placement of metalwork. Before the advent of this technology, serial plain film radiographs were used intra-operatively to confirm verte-bral level and screw position on 2-D images, with no indication of the posi-tion of soft tissues. Pedicle screws were placed blindly, using anatomical landmarks to guide entry point and trajectory. Incorrect placement risks damage to exiting nerve roots inferomedially and to the vertebral artery laterally in the cervical spine. Intra-operative CT quickly delivers 3-D images of the vertebral body and associated soft tissues, enabling metalwork to be guided into position accurately and safely.

FUNCTIONAL NEURONAVIGATION

As tumour resection becomes progressively radical, the importance of delin-eating the interface with healthy and eloquent brain is vital. CT and MR images help identify structural differences between tissue areas, but for the identification of functional areas of brain demarcated by their activity an alternative form of navigation must be employed. Different techniques are used for the identification of both cortical grey matter and its corre-sponding white matter tracts.

Intra-operative electrocortical stimulation maps the surface of cortical motor areas in patients anaesthetized without paralysing agents. Mapping of language areas requires the patient to be woken intra-operatively. These techniques are likely to be superseded by the less invasive imaging based techniques. fMRI and PET map out regional changes in cerebral blood flow and metabolism, respectively. By comparing the distribution of blood flow at rest and during specific tasks, functional areas of brain can be identified.

Diffusion-tensor imaging (DTI) is an emerging MR-based modality which measures the direction of motion of water molecules in axons and myelin sheaths. It is capable of broadly mapping the direction of white matter tracts and can be integrated with grey matter images to reveal eloquent cortex and its corresponding descending fibres.

Modern neuronavigation systems are capable of combining structural imaging with functional imaging, and facilitate resection of a maximal volume of diseased tissue without damaging adjacent healthy brain.

THE O-ARM®

One of the most sophisticated neuronavigation systems currently available is the O-arm®, which is being installed in a growing number of neurosurgical units. It is a mobile 2-D and 3-D intra-operative imaging platform which allows for real-time intra-operative imaging, thereby facilitating intra-operative decision making. It has a very large field of view, and its robotic and sliding door mechanisms facilitate easy and precise intra-operative positioning over the operative site. There are two imaging modes: a 3-D CT mode and a multi-plane 2-D fluoroscopic mode. The field of view provided is three-fold and six-fold larger than that provided by a standard C-arm image intensifier in 2-D and 3-D modes, respectively. The system is also extremely fast, with 3-D images being constructed in under 14 s for standard definition, and under 26 s for high definition.

The O-arm® has many applications in spinal surgery, with the 2-D mode allowing for intra-operative imaging of spinal screw fixations, and the 3-D mode being particularly helpful in guiding instrumentation in the cervical spine. 3-D CT imaging can also be used to facilitate the fixation of maxillofacial injuries. This versatile neuronavigation equipment will have a major impact in the field of functional neurosurgery: the ability to superimpose intra-operative CT images over pre-op MRI images will facilitate electrode placement by allowing trajectories to be checked intra-operatively, and this, in its turn, will significantly reduce the length of surgery by obviating the need for the patient to be transferred to a CT scanner to check final electrode position.

The O-arm® is one of the most useful innovations in neuronavigation in recent years, and is set to become an integral part of the neurosurgical theatre in the near future.

13
Controversies and Evidence in Neurosurgery

Reuben D. Johnson and Jignesh Tailor

CONTENTS

INTRODUCTION

The aim of this chapter is not to review systematically the evidence base in neurosurgery, nor is it to identify every area of controversy in neurosurgery. We have selected a few topics that often crop up in discussions in morning meetings, in theatre, and on the wards. It is hoped that this chapter will give new trainees a basis on which to participate actively in these discussions. Although there are many randomized trials in neurosurgery, it is important to be aware of some of the trials that have influenced the practice of neurosurgery, as they make good points for discussion during theatre, clinic or ward round, and are also often asked about in neurosurgical interviews. Not all such trials can be covered here, but some of the key trials have been outlined in two tables in order to provide useful summaries that will, we hope, help in remembering the key facts. Table 13.1 gives an overview of the key trials that have changed management of neurosurgical patients. When analyzing a randomized controlled trial, be aware of the population, intervention, comparator and outcome (use the acronym PICO to remember this). Table 13.2 gives a summary of ongoing trials, the results of which will be worth looking out for.

PROPHYLACTIC ANTIBIOTICS IN NEUROSURGERY

The use of antibiotics in neurosurgery is widespread yet remains controversial due to the paucity of a solid evidence base. This reflects the difficulties in gathering data in this area of neurosurgery. For example, although in skull fractures with associated CSF leak the incidence of infection may be as high as 25%, the actual incidence of CSF leak is very low. This means that it is extremely difficult to undertake a proper prospective study to compare prophylactic antibiotic regimens with acute treatment of frank infection. The rationale for recommendations regarding the use of prophylactic antibiotics in neurosurgery tends to be based on assessments of the risk of infection, the likely organisms involved, and the penetration of the antibiotic to the site of infection (e.g., CSF penetration across the blood–brain barrier, or penetration of tissues in the surgical field).

The British Society for Antimicrobial Chemotherapy has established working parties to review the evidence on the use of antibiotics in all surgical specialties and its web-pages provide a useful resource of summaries and conclusions regarding antibiotic prophylaxis (www.bsac.org.uk). The working party on neurosurgical infections looked at skull fractures, CSF leaks, and neurosurgical procedures (clean, non-implant surgery; clean–contaminated surgical procedures, e.g., breach of a cranial sinus or naso-/oro-pharynx; CSF and shunt surgery).

Table 13.1. A selection of some of the most important clinical trials.

Clinical trial	Population (P), Intervention (I), Comparator (C) and Outcome (O)	How the result has changed neurosurgical practice

Pickard et al., BMJ 1989; 298:636-642.

| British Aneurysm Nimodipine Trial | P – 554 patients with SAH
I – Nimodipine 60 mg 4 hourly for 21 days
C – Placebo 4 hourly for 21 days
O – Incidence of delayed ischaemic events at 3 months follow-up | Nimodipine significantly reduces the incidence of cerebral, infarction, and is now prescribed routinely in all SAH patients to prevent vasospasm. |

http://www.crash.lshtm.ac.uk/

| Corticosteroid Randomization After Severe Head injury trial (CRASH) | P – 10,008 patients with head injury (GCS 14 or less)
I – 48 hours methylprednisolone infusion
C – 48 hour placebo infusion
O – Death or severe disability at 6 months post-injury | The risk of death or severe disability was significantly higher with corticosteroid treatment, and is therefore not used routinely in current management of head injury. |

http://www.surgery.ox.ac.uk/nvru/isat

| International Subarachnoid Aneurysm Trial (ISAT) | P – 2143 patients with ruptured intracranial aneurysms
I – neurosurgical clipping ($n = 1070$)
C – endovascular coiling ($n = 1073$)
O – death or dependence at 1 year (Rankin score 3–6). Plus, rate of re-bleeding and seizures. | The risk of death or dependence was significantly higher in patients who underwent neurosurgical clipping at 1 year, which has lead to rapid development in endovascular coiling in Europe. Long term follow-up continues. |

Mendelow et al., Lancet 2005; 365: 387–397.

| Surgical Trial in Intracerebral Haemorrhage (STICH) | P – 1033 patients with spontaneous supratentorial intracerebral haemorrhage
I – early surgical evacuation of haematoma
C – initial conservative management
O – Glasgow Outcome Score at 6 months follow-up | A small, non-significant advantage was found for early surgery. However, a large number of patients with spontaneous ICH that underwent early surgery also had intraventricular haemorrhage – a poor prognostic factor. This may have confounded a true difference in outcomes, therefore STICH-II trial is currently underway (see below). |

Table 13.2. Important ongoing clinical trials.

Clinical trial	Population (P), Intervention (I), Comparator (C) and Outcome (O)	How the result has changed neurosurgical practice

http://www.rescueicp.com

| Randomized Evaluation of Surgery with Craniectomy for Uncontrollable Elevation of Intracranial Pressure (RESCUE-ICP) | P – Patients requiring ventilation and ICP monitoring with refractory intracranial hypertension
I – early decompressive craniectomy
C – medical management
O – GOS at discharge and 6 months post-injury | This trial may help to define the role of decompressive craniectomy in management of severe head injuries. |

http://www.stashtrial.com

| SimvasTatin in Aneurysmal Subarachnoid Haemorrhage Trial (STASH) | P – Patients with clinical and radiological diagnosis of SAH from multiple centres, mainly in UK
I – 40mg simvastatin started within 96 hours of ictus, for 3 weeks
C – Placebo (same regime)
O – Death and disability (measured using Rankin Score) at 6 months | The investigators hypothesize that simvastatin reduces the risk of vasospasm following SAH. The results of Phase-II studies are encouraging and some centres have started to use simvastatin as part of the initial management work-up for SAH patients. Watch this space! |

http://www.ncl.ac.uk/stich/

| Surgical Trial in Intracerebral Haemorrhage – II (STICH-II) | P – Patients with spontaneous lobar ICH (excluding IVH)
I – early surgery
C – initial conservation Management
O – Death or disability at 6 months follow-up | Following STICH–I trial (see above) this trial may show a difference in outcome in favour of early surgery for spontaneous lobar ICH. |

SKULL FRACTURES AND CSF LEAK

Up to 25% of patients with CSF leaks associated with base-of-skull fractures will develop infections. The most common organisms causing post-traumatic meningitis are *Pneumococcus* spp. There are certain situations, however, when *Staphylococcus aureus* and Gram −ve bacilli will be causative organisms, namely, in: depressed skull fractures; penetrating brain injuries; patients who have already been on antibiotics for other reasons; and those who have been in hospital for a length of time. The use of prophylactic antibiotics in skull fractures with CSF leak is not supported, due to the paucity of conclusive evidence. However, the situation with penetrating brain injury is somewhat different, as there appears to be a particularly high risk of infection, including meningitis, osteomyelitis and cerebral abscess formation. Although evidence is not available, because appropriate randomized controlled trials have not yet been performed, prophylactic antibiotic use has become widespread routine practice. This seems to be supported by lower rates of infection recorded in studies conducted after World War II, compared with the results of earlier studies (Arabi et al., 2001). Due to the wide spectrum of organisms that appear to be responsible for infection in penetrating brain injury, treatment with broad-spectrum antibiotics tends to be recommended, such as 5 days of co-amoxiclav 1.2 g IV tds, or 5 days cefuroxime 1.5 g IV stat followed by 750 mg IV tds plus metronidazole 500 mg IV tds.

NEUROSURGICAL PROCEDURES

Clean, non-implant surgery

The British Society for Antimicrobial Chemotherapy Working Party concluded that there is a significant amount of evidence to show that antibiotic prophylaxis may be beneficial for clean non-implant surgery. Antibiotics were recommended on the basis of appropriate spectrum of activity (efficacy against likely pathogens: *S. aureus*; other Gram +ve cocci; and Gram −ve bacilli), as well as penetration to the surgical field. An example regimen would be cefuroxime 1.5 g IV at induction of anaesthesia, followed by further 750 mg doses every 3 h during operation. It was concluded that there was no evidence to support prolonging prophylaxis beyond the time of surgery. However, there is no real evidence the other way either, and a commonly used regimen includes two further doses of cefuroxime at 8-h intervals following the first dose at induction.

Clean–contaminated surgery

The British Society for Antimicrobial Chemotherapy Working Party concluded that the case for antibiotic prophylaxis was supported by available evidence, and recommendations included the use of cefuroxime and metronidazole at induction and for the duration of surgery, but no longer.

CSF shunt surgery

The British Society for Antimicrobial Chemotherapy Working Party could not find any evidence that antibiotic prophylaxis is beneficial in shunt surgery. Due to the potentially devastating consequences of shunt infection, however, the large majority of neurosurgeons will elect to use antibiotics. The working party, therefore, proposed that the choice of antibiotic should be based on organisms commonly responsible for shunt infection, i.e., coagulase-negative *Staphylococcus* spp. (90%), *S. aureus* (>20%), and aerobic Gram −ve bacilli (>10%). Theoretically at least, vancomycin and gentamicin would be effective, but neither enters the CSF well from the peripheral circulation, and they would therefore have to be given intraventricularly. It is, however, common for neurosurgeons to soak and prime shunts with gentamicin solution before insertion. Many people also use a cefuroxime regimen to cover external infection from the wound.

Arabi, B, Alden, T, Chesnut R et al.. Antibiotic prophylaxis for penetrating brain injury. J Trauma 2001; 51: S34–S40. This excellent review of the evidence supporting the recommendation to use antibiotic prophylaxis in penetrating brain injury can be viewed on-line at www.neurosurgery.org/trauma/guidelines/.

www.bsac.org.uk/pyxis/ Website summarizing findings of a Working Party of the British Association of Antimicrobial Chemotherapists into Neurosurgical Infection.

ISSUES IN HEAD INJURY

ANTICONULSANTS

The use of anticonvulsants, and of phenytoin in particular, is widespread practice with patients who suffer seizures following traumatic brain injury. More controversial, however, is the use of phenytoin prophylactically to prevent seizures occurring, especially when one has to balance the potentially harmful adverse effects of medication.

Up to 50% of patients suffering a penetrating brain injury will develop seizures. Of these, approximately 10% will show seizures in the first week following injury, and by 2 years 80% of those who are going to fit will have done so (Pruitt, 2001). A seizure occurring in the first week is referred to as an early post-traumatic seizure (EPTS); seizures occurring after this period are referred to as delayed post-traumatic seizures (DPTS). Studies looking at antiepileptic use in brain injury usually consider the effectiveness of anticonvulsants on EPTS and DPTS separately. When considering the use of anticonvulsants to prevent DPTS it is important to realise that 95% of patients suffering penetrating brain injury will remain seizure free if they have not suffered a seizure in the first 3 years (Weiss et al., 1986).

The published evidence is limited and conflicting. Where trials have been conducted there is considerable disagreement regarding the validity of the methodology. For a good recent example of two conflicting opinions, read the correspondence between Professors Chang and Lowenstein of Harvard Medical School and Professor Latronico of the University of Brescia, Italy (Chang and Lowenstein, 2003). Basically, there is one body of opinion suggesting that phenytoin is effective in reducing EPTS but not DPTS, and another body of opinion that holds that phenytoin is lacking in efficacy in both situations. There are even two conflicting trials that back up each point of view. Temkin et al. (1990) undertook a randomized, double-blind study of 404 patients at risk of post-traumatic seizures; 208 received phenytoin within 24 h of injury and 196 received placebo. A 3.6% incidence of EPTS was reported in the phenytoin group, compared to 14.2% in the placebo group. No effect on DPTS was found. The authors concluded that phenytoin is beneficial against EPTS only in the first week after severe head injury. This is in contradiction to the finding of an earlier, similar trial undertaken by Young et al. (1973) which involved 244 patients, and in which no benefit was found for phenytoin in either EPTS or DPTS.

It would appear from the evidence so far that if there is any benefit from phenytoin it will be only in EPTS, and so administration for a longer period of time would not be necessary. However, the existing evidence is there to help in the decision-making process, and it is appropriate, when considering anticonvulsants in individual cases, to take account of the extent to which their situation resembles those of patients included in the existing trials. Individual Consultants working side-by-side within the same neuro-surgical unit may differ in their practice with regard to prophylactic pheny-toin. It is an interesting exercise to enquire as to their reasons, as they will have a wealth of clinical experience which will have shaped their practice. So far, there is little evidence concerning the degree to which the nature of penetrating brain injury influences the risk of post-traumatic seizure, e.g., the site of cortical injury, the presence of a foreign body, or infection. This does not mean to say that such factors are not relevant, but only that there just has not been a study big enough to find any answers.

Chang BS, Lowenstein DG. Practice parameter: antiepileptic drug prophylaxis in severe trau-matic brain injury. Neurology 2003; 60: 10–16 (See also associated correspondence).

Pruit B. Antiseizure prophylaxis for penetrating brain injury. J Trauma 2001; 51: S41–S44.

Temkin NR, Dikmen SS, Wilensky AJ, Keihm J, Chabal S, Winn HR. A randomised, double-blinded study of phenytoin for the prevention of post-traumatic seizures. N Engl J Med 1990; 8: 497–502.

Weiss GH, Salazar AM, Vance SC, Grafman JH, Jabbain B. Predicting posttraumatic epilepsy in penetrating head injury. Arch Neurol 1986; 43: 771–773.

Young B, Rapp RP, Norton JA, Haack D, Tibbs PA, Bean JR. Failure of prophylactically admin-istered phenytoin to prevent early posttraumatic seizures. J Neurosurg 1983; 58: 231–235.

STEROIDS

A comprehensive review of randomized trials on the use of steroids in head injury was undertaken by Alderson and Roberts (1997) who found that, even when all patient data from the trials were combined, the numbers of patients involved was only a little over 2000, and there seemed to be only a statistically nonsignificant 2% reduction in mortality with the use of steroids. Nevertheless, a 2% reduction in mortality would represent a large number of lives saved in view of the millions of deaths from severe head injury that occur each year. This was the incentive for the subsequent CRASH trial, a randomized placebo-controlled trial of intravenous steroids in adults with head injury. The trial, involving 9673 patients, was completed in 2005; the 6-month outcomes were given by Edwards et al. (2005) and showed a significantly higher risk of death, and a nonsignificantly higher risk of death or severe disability, with corticosteroids than with placebo. The investigators concluded that corticosteroids should not be routinely administered in the treatment of head injury. Notwithstanding the CRASH trial results, steroid use will undoubtedly be discussed when head injury patients are transferred in, and opinions may differ greatly. It is pertinent to consider the implications of reduced mortality in severe head injury. One step up in outcome from death is severe morbidity. Is death really always the worst outcome? If the use of steroids in severe head injury is to be accepted by neurosurgeons, this should be based on studies showing a reduction in severe morbidity.

Alderson P and Roberts I. Corticosteroids in acute traumatic brain injury: systematic review of randomised controlled trials. Br Med J 1997; 314: 1855–1859.

Edwards P, Arango M, Balica L et al. Final results of MRC CRASH, a randomised placebo-controlled trial of intravenous corticosteroids in adults with head injury – outcomes at 6 months. Lancet 2005; 9475: 1957–1959.

THIOPENTONE TO CONTROL ICP IN SEVERE HEAD INJURY

The use of barbiturates, such as thiopentone, to control intracranial pressure (ICP) remains controversial, particularly because their administration prolongs the stay of severely brain-damaged patients in the intensive care unit (ICU), without necessarily improving their clinical outcome. It was shown that the administration of barbiturates is effective in lowering ICP (Shapiro et al., 1979). Although it is widely accepted that control of ICP improves survival and outcome in severe head injury, there is conflicting evidence that the use of high-dose barbiturates achieves this aim (Rea and Lockswold, 1983; Ward et al., 1985).

Rea GL, Rockswold GL. Barbiturate therapy in uncontrolled hypertension. Neurosurgery 1983; 12: 401–404.

Shapiro HM, Wyte SR, Loeser J. Barbiturate augmented hypothermia for reduction of persistent intracranial hypertension. J Neurosurg 1979; 40: 90–100.

Ward JD, Becker DP, Miller JD et al. Failure of prophylactic barbiturate coma in the treatment of severe head injury. J Neurosurg 1985; 62: 383–388.

EARLY DECOMPRESSIVE CRANIECTOMY

Decompressive craniectomy is often performed in severe head injury as a 'last resort' for the treatment of uncontrolled raised intracranial pressure. A bone flap is removed and the dura opened to give the swollen brain more space. Although this reduces intracranial pressure and improves cerebral perfusion pressure, its effect on neurological outcome is controversial. There is some concern that the operation may not improve the favourable outcome of patients with a good prognosis, but merely shifts the outcome from death to a persistent vegetative state or severe disability in patients with poor prognosis. Previous studies (mostly class II and III) are inconclusive, demonstrate a wide range of clinical outcomes, and provide no clear consensus regarding the indication for the operation (Hutchinson et al, 2005). The RESCUEicp trial is a randomized trial comparing medical management with decompressive craniectomy for the management of raised intracranial pressure in patients with severe head injury refractory to first-line medical treatment. The primary end-point of the trial is the Glasgow outcome score (GOS) at discharge and 6 months; however the time in ICU and hospital, and quality of life will also be compared. Further details of the trial can be found on the web (www.rescueicp.com). The trial is currently recruiting patients and will undoubtedly shed light on the role of decompressive craniectomy in head injury in the near future.

Hutchinson P, Menon D, Kirkpatrick PJ. Decompressive craniectomy in traumatic brain injury – time for randomised trials? Acta Neurochir 2005; 147 (1): 1-3

ISSUES IN SUBARACHNOID HAEMORRHAGE

NIMODIPINE TO PREVENT SECONDARY CEREBRAL ISCHAEMIA

Secondary ischaemia is a significant cause of poor outcome in subarachnoid haemorrhage (SAH), and may be due to vasospasm. A double-blind, placebo-controlled trial involving 554 patients (Pickard et al., 1980) found that the calcium antagonist, nimodipine, seemed to be effective in reducing cerebral infarction and the incidence of poor outcome at 3 months in SAH patients. A Cochrane review (Rinkel et al., 2002) looked at the evidence gathered subsequently from 11 trials and concluded that it favoured the use of nimodipine. However, the evidence is only for oral nimodipine given 4-hourly, and not for IV regimens. In addition, the Cochrane review indicated that the efficacy of calcium antagonists might not be as clear-cut for patients with established ischaemia or with a poor initial grade of SAH. Further studies may reveal improved dosing regimens and consider the efficacy of calcium antagonists other than nimodipine.

Pickard JD, Murray GD, Illingworth R et al. The effect of oral nimodipine on cerebral infarction and outcome after subarachnoid haemorrhage. Br Med J 1989; 298: 636–640.

Rinkel GJ, Feigh VL, Alagra A, Vermeulen M, Van Gijn J. Calcium antagonists for anuerysmal subarachnoid haemorrhage. Cochrane Database Syst Rev 2002; 4: CD000277.

ENDOVASCULAR COILING *VERSUS* SURGERY

Good clinical trials are rumoured to be rare in surgery. However, you should be aware of one particularly good neurosurgical trial that was reported recently. This is the International Subarachnoid Aneurysm Trial (ISAT) (International Subarachnoid Haemorrhage Collaborative Group, 2002) which compared the safety and efficacy of endovascular coiling of aneurysms with that of surgical clipping. This randomized, multicentre trial was undertaken in Europe, and 2143 patients were enrolled. The ISAT group reported that coiling appeared to be safe and that its efficacy was significantly better than that of surgical clipping in terms of survival free of disability at 1 year. Follow-up of patients in the trial is still under way. The trial has not been without its critics, however. Some observers have argued that, although the ISAT group showed that coiling was safe compared to clipping, the evidence was not as convincing for efficacy (Leung et al., 2003). Others have argued that there is an expertise bias in favour of endovascular interventionalists (Britz et al., 2003). The response of the ISAT group to such criticisms can be read in the literature (Molyneaux and Kerr, 2003). Further follow-up of data in the ISAT trial are due to be published in the near future and will be well worth looking out for.

Britz GW, Newell DW, West A, Lam A. The ISAT trial. Lancet 2003; 361: 431–432.

International Subarachnoid Haemorrhage Collaborative Group. International Subarachnoid Aneurysm Trial (ISAT) of neurosurgical clipping *versus* endovascular coiling in 2143 patients with ruptured intracranial aneurysms: a randomised trial. Lancet 2002; 360: 1267–1274.

Leung CHS, Poon WS, Yu LM. The ISAT trial. Lancet 2003; 361: 430–431.

Molyneux A, Kerr A. The ISAT trial. Lancet 2003; 361: 432.

PERIOPERATIVE ANTICONVULSANT PROPHYLAXIS

Although the administration of prophylactic anticonvulsant medication has been accepted practice for aneurysmal surgery for many years, the benefits of these medications need to be balanced against the risk of adverse reactions. A retrospective study (Baker et al., 1995) found that the incidence of seizures following craniotomy for aneurysm repair was low, and it was concluded that the administration of prophylactic phenytoin was necessary only for the first 7 days postoperatively. There seems to be a paucity of strong evidence for the prolonged use of prophylactic anticonvulsants in SAH.

Baker CJ, Prestigiacomo CJ, Solomon RA. Short-term perioperative anticonvulsant prophylaxis for the surgical treatment of low-risk patients with intracranial aneurysms. Neurosurgery 1995; 37: 863–871.

TIMING OF SURGERY FOR SUBARACHNOID HAEMORRHAGE

The timing of subarachnoid surgery is one of the most contentious issues in neurosurgery. In some cases, the presence of a large, life-threatening clot demands early craniotomy. Indeed, it can be argued that, on theoretical grounds, there are good reasons to operate in the first 2–3 days following rupture, e.g., the risk of re-bleeding will be reduced, and protection of the aneurysm allows for more aggressive treatment of vasospasm. However, there are equally good arguments against early surgery, e.g., the amount of blood and brain oedema present immediately after a bleed makes surgery more difficult (due to difficulty retracting the parenchyma) and operative mortality is higher. Although there have been a number of studies looking at this issue, there is still no consensus (Milhorat and Krautheim 1986; Kassel et al., 1990; de Gans et al., 2002).

de Gans K, Nieuwkamp DJ, Rinkel GJ, Algra A. Timing of aneurysm surgery in subarachnoid hemorrhage: a systematic review of the literature. Neurosurgery 2002; 50: 336–340.

Kassell NF, Torner JC, Haley EC Jr, Jane JA, Adams HP, Kongable GL. The International Cooperative Study on the Timing of Aneurysm Surgery. Part 1: Overall management results. J Neurosurg 1990; 73: 18–36.

Kassell NF, Torner JC, Jane JA. The international cooperative study on the timing of aneurysm surgery. Part 2: Surgical results. J Neurosurg 1990; 73: 37–47.

Milhorat TH, Krautheim M. Results of early and delayed operations for ruptured intracranial aneurysms in two series of 100 consequetive patients. Surg Neurol 1986; 26: 123–128.

MANAGEMENT OF UNRUPTURED ANEURYSMS

The International Study of Unruptured Intracranial Aneurysms (ISUIA) was the first large-scale prospective study to look at the natural history of unruptured aneurysms as well as the risks of treatment of unruptured aneurysms. A total of 4060 patients from 61 centres world-wide were included in the study. The study concluded that aneurysmal rupture rate is related to the size and location of the aneurysm, and that even for aneurysms <7mm, the risk is increased with previous SAH from a separate aneurysm. These factors, coupled with the morbidity/mortality data, allow neurosurgeons to make an informed choice on whether to operate or not. In general, the risk of rupture for a particular aneurysm over the patient's remaining lifetime can be compared with the mortality/morbidity risk. The ISUIA study is the best natural history study to date. Although there have been criticisms regarding selection bias, the ISUIA has had a profound impact on the decision to treat unruptured aneurysms.

International Study of Unruptured Intracranial Aneurysms Investigators. Unruptured intracranial aneurysms: natural history, clinical outcome, and risks of surgical and endovascular treatment. Lancet 2003; 362: 103–10

ISSUES IN THE SURGICAL MANAGEMENT OF STROKE

DECOMPRESSIVE SURGERY FOR MALIGNANT CEREBRAL ARTERY INFARCTION

Malignant MCA infarction (MMI) is associated with a mortality of 80%. Since 2000, three European trials have addressed the role of decompressive surgery in these patients: the DECIMAL trial (decompressive craniectomy in malignant MCA infarction) performed in France; the DESTINY trial (decompresive surgery for the treatment of malignant infarction of the MCA) performed in Germany; and the HAMLET trial (hemicraniectomy after MCA infarction with life-treatening edema trial) performed in the Netherlands. Although HAMLET was still ongoing, a pooled analysis of these three trial was published in 2007. The final results of HAMLET have been published in 2009. In addition, a North American trial, the HeaDDFIRST trial (hemicraniectomy and durotomy on deterioration from infarction-related swelling trial), was carried out between 2000 and 2003, although this was only ever published in abstract form. Although the pooled analysis appeared to show that early decompressive surgery for MMI reduces mortality and increases the number of patients with a favourable outcome, this conclusion has been severely criticized. The definition of a favourable outcome included patients who were left with moderately severe disability and many people would not regard this as a favourable outcome. There is still widespread variation in the surgical management of MMI, and the decision to operate is often based on the individual experiences of the surgeons and stroke physicians involved, rather than on any sound evidence base.

Vahedi, K, Hofmeijer J, Juettler E et al. for the DECIMAL, DESTINY and HAMLET investigators. Early decompressive surgery in malignant infarction of the middle cerebral artery: a pooled analysis of three randomised trials. Lancet Neurol 2007; 6: 215–222

Carandang RA, Krieger DW. Decompressive hemicraniectomy and durotomy for malignant middle cerebral artery infarction. Neurocrit Care 2008; 8: 286–289.

SURGERY FOR SPONTANEOUS INTRACEREBRAL HAEMATOMAS

The International Surgical Trial in Intracerebral Haematoma (STICH) is the largest randomized controlled trial evaluating the role of early surgery in the management of intracerebral haematomas, and included 1033 patients. The study was headed by Professor Mendelow from Newcastle General Hospital and was funded by the Medical Research Council (UK). The study concluded that there is no overall benefit from early surgery *versus* initial conservative treatment for spontaneous supratentorial haematomas. Subgroup analysis showed that a favourable outcome was more likely with early surgery for superficially-based lesions (≤ 1 cm from cortical surface) with a 29% relative benefit, but this difference was not statistically significant. A further trial, STICH II, is now under way to elucidate further the role of surgery for more superficially based lesions.

Mendelow AD, Gregson BA, Fernandes HN et al. for the STICH investigators. Early surgery *versus* initial conservative treatment in patients with spontaneous supratentorial intracerebral haematomas in the International Surgical Trial in Intracerebral Haemorrhage (STICH): a randomised trial. Lancet 2005; 365: 387–397
Mendelow AD, Unterberg A. Surgical treatment of intracerebral haemorrhage. Curr Opin Crit Care 2007; 13: 169-174.

ISSUES IN NEURO-ONCOLOGY

SURGERY FOR A SINGLE BRAIN METASTASIS

There have been three randomized trials evaluating the role of surgical resection in the treatment of solitary brain metastasis. All three trials compared surgical resection plus radiotherapy *versus* radiotherapy alone. Two out of the three trials found surgery plus radiotherapy to be superior to radiotherapy alone for single cerebral metastasis. All three trials have been criticised for different reasons, and there is ongoing controversy as to whether there is a role for resection of a solitary brain metastasis. Discussions of these patients at neuro-oncology multidisciplinary team meetings can be very interesting indeed.

Patchell RA, Tibbs PA, Walsh JW et al. A randomized trial of surgery in the treatment of single metastases to the brain. N Eng J Med 1990; 322: 494–500.
Vecht CJ, Haaxma-Reiche H, Noordijk EM et al. Treatment of single brain metastasis: radiotherapy alone or combined with neurosurgery? Ann Neurol 1993; 33: 583–590.
Mintz AH, Kestle J, Rathbone MP et al. A randomized trial to assess the efficacy of surgery in addition to radiotherapy in patients with a single cerebral metastasis. Cancer 1996; 78: 1470–1476.

EXTENT OF RESECTION FOR MALIGNANT GLIOMA

There is consideratble debate as to whether the extent of resection of malignant glioma has any effect on outcome. The most frequently quoted study is a large retrospective analysis of 92 patients from the Washington Medical Center in Seattle, which concluded that there is a survival advantage from increased resection (Keles et al., 1999). Furthermore, there has been one randomized trial of biopsy *versus* debulking surgery, and this showed a moderate survival advantage of debulking (Vuorinen et al., 2003)

Keles GE, Anderson B, Berger MS. The effect of extent of resection on time to tumor progression and survival in patients with glioblastoma mulitforme of the cerebral hemisphere. Cancer 1999; 74: 1784–1791.
Vuorinen V, Hinkka S, Farkilla M, Jasskelainen J. Debulking or biopsy of malignant glioma in elderly people – a randomized study. Acta Neurochir (Wein) 2003; 145: 5–10.

CARMUSTINE WAFERS FOR MALIGNANT GLIOMAS

Three randomized, controlled trials have been carried out to evaluate the effect of local administration of carmustine wafers (Gliadel) to the tumour site in patients with malignant gliomas. The largest trial found a 2-month survival advantage with carmustine wafers applied to the resection cavity at first operation.

Brem H, Piantadosi S, Burger PC et al. for the Polymer-Brain Tumor Treatment Group. Lancet 1995; 345: 1008–1012.
Westphal M, Hilt DC, Bortey E et al. A phase 3 trial of local chemotherapy with biodegradable carmustine (BCNU) wafers (Gliadel wafers) in patients with primary malignant glioma. Neuro-Oncology 2003; 5: 79–88.
Westphal M, Ram Z, Riddle V et al. Gliadel wafer in initial surgery for malignant glioma: long-term follow-up of a multi-center controlled trial. Acta Neurochir (Wein) 2006; 148: 269–275.

ISSUES IN SPINAL SURGERY
STEROIDS FOR SPINAL INJURY

Several clinical trials have been done to evaluate the use of steroids in spinal cord injury. However, this treatment modality remains controversial and practice differs between clinicians and centres.

A Cochrane review of the evidence (Bracken, 2000) found that too few studies had been conducted in this area for definitive conclusions to be reached, but that a meta-analysis of three trials (one in North America, one in Japan, and one in France) had shown some apparent benefit for methyl prednisolone. However, there has been much discussion in the literature regarding the methodology of these trials. Improved outcome in motor function was seen at 1 year, provided that methyl prednisolone was given within 8 h of injury and in the following regimen: (1) 30 mg/kg bolus; (2) an infusion of 5.4 mg/kg/h for a further 23 h. It was also possible that further motor improvement might occur if infusion was continued for a total of 48 h. A more recent review found that, although neurological improvement was seen with methyl prednisolone, there was no effect on overall mortality (Spencer and Bazarian, 2003). All reviewers indicate that further studies are required to establish the efficacy of corticosteroids in spinal cord injury, and appropriate treatment regimens for their use.

Bracken MB. Steroids for acute spinal injury. Cochrane Database Syst Rev 2000; 2: CD001046.
Spencer MT, Bazarian JJ. Are corticosteroids effective in traumatic spinal cord injury? Ann Emerg Med 2003; 41: 410–413.

TIMING OF SURGERY FOR CAUDA EQUINA SYNDROME

Although there is no prospective randomized trial evaluating the timing of surgery for cauda equina syndrome (CES), published case series have strongly supported the view that CES is a diagnostic and surgical emergency, and that early surgery results in a better outcome than delayed surgery (O'Laoire et al., 1981, Shapiro, 2000). Two meta-analyses of published case series have been carried out, and these support the view that timing of surgery does affect outcome (Ahn et al., 2000; Todd, 2005; Jerwood and Todd, 2006).

However, this view has received vehement opposition from some quarters (Gleave and McFarlane, 2002; Findlay, 2008). The timing of surgery for CES continues, therefore, to be an extremely controversial issue.

Ahn UM, Ahn NU, Buchowski MS et al. Cauda equina syndrome secondary to lumbar disc herniation. A meta-analysis of surgical outcomes. Spine 2000; 25: 1515–1522.

Findlay G. Meta-analysis and the timing of cauda equina surgery. B J Neurosurg 2008; 22: 137–138.

Gleave JR, MacFarlane R. Cauda equina syndrome: what is the relationship between timing of surgery and outcome. B J Neurosurg 2002; 16: 325–328.

Jerwood D, Todd NV. Reanalysis of the timing of cauda equina surgery. Br J Neurosurg. 2006; 20: 178–179.

O'Laoire SA, Crockard HA, Thomas DG. Prognosis for sphinctor recovery after operation for cauda equina compression owing to lumbar disc prolapse. BMJ 1981; 282: 1852–1854.

Shapiro S. Medical realities of cauda equina syndrome secondary to lumbar disc herniation. Spine. 2000; 25: 348–51.

Todd NV. Cauda equina syndrome: the timing of surgery probably does influence outcome. B J Neurosurg 2005; 19: 301–306.

14
Commonly Used Scoring Systems in Neurosurgery

W. Adriaan Liebenberg and Reuben D. Johnson

CONTENTS

The Glasgow Coma Scale
The Glasgow Outcome Scale
WFNS grade of subarachnoid haemorrhage
Fisher grade of CT findings in subarachnoid haemorrhage
Karnofsky score
MRC score for muscle strength assessment

THE GLASGOW COMA SCALE

Table 14.1 is a modified version of the Glasgow Coma Scale (GCS). See also the discussion of the GCS in Chapter 4 (p. 54), which deals with neurosurgical history and examination.

Table 14.1. The Modified Glasgow Coma Scale.

Score	Eye opening (max = 4)	Verbal response (max = 5)	Motor response (max = 6)
6	–	–	Obeys
5	–	Orientated	Localizes
4	Spontaneous	Confused	Withdraws
3	To speech	Inappropriate	Flexion (decorticate)
2	To pain	Incomprehensible	Extension (decerebrate)
1	None	None	None

Teasdale G, Jennett B. Assessment of coma and impaired consciousness: a practical scale. Lancet 1974; ii: 81–84.

THE GLASGOW OUTCOME SCALE

Table 14.2 is a modified summary of the Glasgow Outcome Scale (GOS), which was designed for the assessment of outcome in head injuries. The GOS is a valuable and established research tool. When critically evaluating new treatment modalities for head injury that are reported to produce improvements in the GOS, it is necessary to consider exactly what that means for the patient. For example, a treatment modality might be shown to improve the GOS in 90% of patients; however, if the improvement equates to improvements from a GOS of 1 to 2, i.e., from death to a persistent vegetative state, then it is worth considering the implications for the patient. Is death always the worst outcome?

Table 14.2. The Glasgow Outcome Scale (modified).

Score	Description of patient
5	Normal life
4	Mild disability, able to perform basic activities of daily life independently, but not able to resume previously normal life
3	Severely disabled and dependent
2	Persistent vegetative state
1	Death

Jennett B, Bond M. The assessment of outcome after severe brain damage: a practical scale. Lancet 1975; i: 480–484.

WFNS GRADE OF SUBARACHNOID HAEMORRHAGE

The World Federation of Neurological Surgeons (WFNS) grading scale (Table 14.3) is a six-point (0 to 5) scale for rating the effects of subarachnoid haemorrhage in terms of GCS score and the presence or absence of focal deficit.

Table 14.3. The World Federation of Neurological Surgeons (WFNS) grading scale for subarachnoid haemorrhage.

WFNS grade	GCS	Focal deficit (aphasia, hemiparesis)
0 (unruptured aneurysm)	–	–
1	15	None
2	13–14	None
3	13–14	Present
4	7–12	None or present
5	3–6	None or present

Drake C G. Report of World Federation of Neurological Surgeons Committee on a universal subarachnoid haemorrhage grading scale. J Neurosurg 1988; 68: 985–986.

FISHER GRADE OF CT FINDINGS IN SUBARACHNOID HAEMORRHAGE

A poor Fisher grade (Table 14.4) correlates with increased risk of vasospasm.

Table 14.4. The Fisher scale for grading CT findings in subarachnoid haemorrhage.

Fisher grade	Blood on CT
1	None detected
2	Diffuse or vertical layers[a] <1 mm thick
3	Localized clot or vertical layer >1 mm thick
4	Intracerebral or intraventricular clot

[a] Vertical layers refers to subarachnoid spaces, e.g., intrahemisphere fissure.

Fisher C M, Kistler J P, Davis J M. Relation of cerebral vasospasm to subarachnoid haemorrhage visualized by CT scanning. Neurosurgery 1980; 6: 1–9.

MRC SCORE FOR MUSCLE STRENGTH ASSESSMENT

Table 14.5. The MRC scale for grading muscle strength.

Grade	Strength
0	No contraction
1	Flicker
2	Moves if gravity eliminated
3	Gravity overcome
4	Moves against resistance
5	Normal strength

KARNOFSKY SCORE

The Karnofsky score (Table 14.6) was devised as a clinical and research tool to grade the functional status in cancer patients. The maximum and best score is 100, which implies normal functioning. Lower scores imply varying degrees of symptomatology, disability and sickness. The lowest score is 0 and implies death.

Table 14.6. The Karnofsky performance score.

Condition and score	Comments

A. Able to carry on normal activity and to work. No special care needed

100	Normal, no complaints, no evidence of disease.
90	Able to carry on normal activity, minor signs or symptoms of disease.
80	Normal activity with effort, some signs or symptoms of disease.

B. Unable to work. Able to live at home, care for most personal needs
A varying degree of assistance is needed.

70	Cares for self. Unable to carry on normal activity or to do active work.
60	Requires occasional assistance, but is able to care for most of own needs.
50	Disease may be progressing rapidly. Requires considerable assistance and frequent medical care.

C. Unable to care for self. Requires equivalent of institutional or hospital care.

40	Disabled. Requires special care and assistance.
30	Severely disabled, hospitalization is indicated although death is not imminent.
20	Hospitalization necessary, very sick, active supportive treatment necessary.
10	Moribund, fatal processes progressing rapidly.
0	Dead.

Karnofsky DA, Burchenal JH. The clinical evaluation of chemotherapeutic agents in cancer. In: Macleod CM, ed. Evaluation of chemotherapy agents. New York: Columbia University Press, 1949: 191–205.
www.acsu.buffalo.edu/~drstall/assessmenttools.html

FURTHER READING

Crockard A, Hayward R, Hoff JT, eds. *Neurosurgery: the Scientific Basis of Clinical Practice*, 3rd edn. Oxford: Blackwell Science, 2000.

Greenberg MS. *Handbook of Neurosurgery*, 6th edn. Berlin: Thieme, 2006.

Jennett B, Lindsay KW. *An Introduction to Neurosurgery*, 5th edn. London: Butterworth Heinemann, 1994.

Kaye AH. *Essential Neurosurgery*, 3rd edn. Malden: Blackwell Publishing, 2005.

Lindsay KW, Bone I. *Neurology and Neurosurgery Illustrated*, 4th edn. Edinburgh: Churchill Livingstone, 2004.

Moore AJ, Newell DW, eds. *Neurosurgery: Principles and Practice*. Berlin: Springer Verlag, 2005.

Patten J. *Neurological Differential Diagnosis*, 2nd edn. Berlin: Springer Verlag, 1996, corr. 2nd printing 1998.

Rengachary SS, Ellenbogen RG. *Principles of Neurosurgery*, 2nd edn. London: Mosby, 2005.

Tindall GT, Cooper PR, Barrow DL, eds. *Practice of Neurosurgery*. London: Lippincott, Williams & Wilkins, 1996

Winn HR, ed. *Youman's Neurological Surgery*, 5th edn. New York: W. B. Saunders, 2003.

ABBREVIATIONS

A&E	Accident and emergency
ACA	Anterior cerebral artery
Acomm	Anterior communicating artery
ACTH	Adreocorticotrophic hormone
ADC	Apparent diffusion coefficient
ADH	Antidiuretic hormone
AF	Atrial fibrillation
AMT	Abbreviated mental test
AP	Anteroposterior
ASDH	Acute subdural haemorrhage/haematoma
ATLS	Advanced trauma life support
AVM	Arteriovenous malformation
BA	Basilar artery
BIH	Benign intracranial hypertension
cACA(A2)	Contralateral anterior cerebral artery A2 segment
CBF	Cerebral blood flow
CBV	Cerebral blood volume
CCrISP	Care of the critically ill surgical patient
CEA	Carcinoembryonic antigen
CES	Cauda equine syndrome
CMR	Cerebral metabolic rate
CNS	Central nervous system
Coag screen	Coagulation screening
CPP	Cerebral perfusion pressure
CRASH	Corticosteroid randomisation after significant head injury
CRP	C-reactive protein
CSDH	Chronic subdural haematoma
CSF	Cerebrospinal fluid
CSW	Cerebral salt wasting
CT	Computerized tomography
CTA	CT angiography
CVA	Cerebrovascular accident
CVP	Central venous pressure
CXR	Chest X-ray
DDAVP	1-d-amino-8-D-arginine vasopressin
DECIMAL	Decompressive craniectomy in malignant MCA infarction
DESTINY	Decompressive surgery for the treatment of malignant infarction of the MCA
DI	Diabetes insipidus
DIND	Delayed ischaemic neurological deficit
DNET	Dysembryoplastic neuroectodermal tumours
DPTS	Delayed post-traumatic seizure
DTI	Diffusion-tensor imaging
DVT	Deep-vein thrombosis
DWI	Diffusion weighted imaging
DWM	Dandy-Walker malformation
EAM	External auditory meatus

ECF	Extra cellular fluid
ECG	Electrocardiogram
EDH	Extradural haemorrhage/haematoma
EEG	Electroencephalogram
EICA	Extracranial internal carotid artery
EMG	Electromyography
EPTS	Early post-traumatic seizure
ESR	Erythrocyte sedimentation rate
ET	Endotracheal
ETV	Endoscopic third ventriculostomy
EVD	External ventricular drain
Ex	Examination
FBC	Full blood count
FiO_2	Fractional inspired oxygen concentration
FLAIR	Fluid attenuated inverse ratio
FSH	Follicle-stimulating hormone
G&S	Group and save
GBM	Glioblastoma multiforme
GCS	Glasgow Coma Scale
GH	Growth hormone
GOS	Glasgow outcome scale
HAMLET	Hemicraniectomy after MC infarction with life-threatening edema trial
β-HCG	Human chorionic gonadotrophin
HDU	High-dependency unit
HeaDDFIRST	Hemicraniectomy and durotomy on deterioration from infarction-related swelling trial
Hx	History
iACA(A2)	Ispilateral anterior cerebral artery A2 segment
ICA	Internal carotid artery
ICP	Intracranial pressure
ICU	Intensive care unit
IgF1	Immunoglobulin F1
IIH	Idiopathic intracranial hypertension
INR	International normalized ratio
ISAT	International Subarachnoid Aneurysm Trial
ISUIA	International Study of Unruptured Intercranial Aneurysm
IQ	Intelligence quotient
IV	Intravenous
IVH	Intraventricular haemorrhage
LAICA	Left anterior inferior cerebellar artery
LAT	Locum Appointment for Training
LFT	Liver function tests
LH	Luteinizing hormone
LICA	Left internal carotid artery
LP	Lumbar puncture
LPICA	Left posterior inferior cerebellar artery
LR	Lindgaard ratio
LVA	Left vertebral artery
MAP	Mean arterial pressure

MCA	Middle cerebral artery
MDT	Multidisciplinary team
MI	Myocardial infarction
MMI	Malignant MCA infarction
MMSE	Mini mental state examination
MRI	Magnetic resonance imaging
MRA	Magnetic resonance angiography
MRC	Medical Research Council
MRI	Magnetic resonance imaging
MRS	Magnetic resonance spectroscopy
NAA	N-acetyl aspartate
NAI	Non-accidental injury
NBM	Nil by mouth
NF1	Neurofibromatosis type 1
NF2	Neurofibromatosis type 2
NICU	Neuro-intensive care unit
NSAID	Non-steroidal anti-inflammatory drug
Obs	Observations
ophth.a	Ophthalmic artery
PCNSL	Primary CNS lymphomas
PCO_2	Partial pressure of carbon dioxide
Pcomm	Posterior communicating artery
PE	Pulmonary embolism
PET	Positron emission tomography
PICU	Paediatric intensive care unit
PNET	Primitive neuroectodermal tumour
PR	Per rectum
PSA	Prostate-specific antigen
PT	Prothrombin time
PTC	Pseudotumour cerebri
PXA	Pleomorphic xanthoastrocytoma
RESCUicp	Randomized Evaluation of Surgery with Craniectomy for Uncontrollable Elevation of Intra-Cranial Pressure
RICA	Right internal carotid artery
RPCA	Right posterior cerebellar artery
RSCA	Right superior cerebellar artery
RTA	Road traffic accident
RVA	Right vertebral artery
SAH	Subarachnoid haemorrhage
Sats	Haemaglobin oxygen saturation
SCIWORA	Spinal cord injury without radiological abnormality
SDH	Subdural haemorrhage
SEGA	Subependymal giant cell astrocytoma
SHO	Senior House Officer
SIADH	Syndrome of inappropriate antidiuretic hormone secretion
SM	Spetzler-Martin
SOS	Site of surgery
SpR	Specialist Registrar
ST1–3	Specialist Trainee years 1–3
STICH	International Surgical Trial in Intracerebral Haematoma

TCD	Transcranial doppler
TE	Time to echo
TR	Time to relaxation
TEDs	Thromboembolic-deterrent stockings
U & E	Urea and electrolytes
VP	Ventriculoperitoneal
WCC	White cell count
WFNS	World Federation of Neurological Surgeons
X-match	Cross match

NOTES

NOTES